THE LITTLE

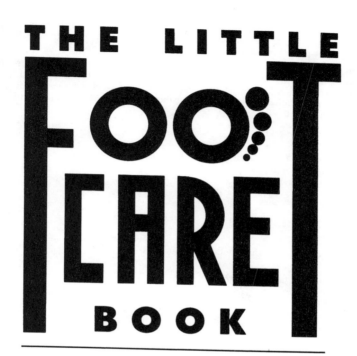

FOOT CARE BOOK

ERIKA DILLMAN

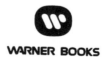

WARNER BOOKS

A Time Warner Company

The information (advice/program) in this book is not intended to be a substitute for medical advice. You are advised to consult with your health care professional with regard to all matters relating to your health, and in particular regarding matters which may require diagnosis or medical attention. If you have heart disease or diabetes, some of the recommendations in this book may not be for you.

Warner Books, Inc., 1271 Avenue of the Americas, New York, NY 10020
Visit our Web site at www.twbookmark.com
Printed in the United States of America

 A Time Warner Company

First Printing: November 2000
10 9 8 7 6 5 4 3 2 1

Library of Congress Cataloging-in-Publication Data

Dillman, Erika.
    The little foot care book / by Erika Dillman.
      p. cm.
    Includes index.
    ISBN 0-446-67626-8
    1. Foot—Care and hygiene—Popular works. 2. Foot—Wounds and injuries—Treatment—Popular works. 3. Foot—Massage—Popular works. I. Title.

RD563.D53 2000
617.5'85—dc21   00-039898

Cover design by Rachel McClain
Book design and text composition by L&G McRee
Text illustrations by Doug Keith
Text illustration on page 63 Erika Dillman

For my grandmother,
Hanna Anderson

Acknowledgments

I'd like to thank the following people for generously sharing with me their time, knowledge, and expertise:

My agent, Anne Depue, for her support and guidance.

All of the medical professionals with whom I consulted throughout this project: Dr. Pierce Scranton Jr., M.D., orthopedic surgeon; Dr. Cherise Dyal, M.D., chief, Division of Foot and Ankle Surgery, Montefiore Medical Center, and assistant professor of orthopedic surgery at Albert Einstein College of Medicine; Dr. Stephen F. Conti, M.D., orthopedic surgeon, chair of the American Orthopaedic Foot and Ankle Society (AOFAS) Public Education Committee, chief, Division of Foot and Ankle Surgery, University of Pittsburgh School of Medicine; Dr. Pam Colman, D.P.M., podiatrist, and director of health affairs for the American Podiatric Medical Association (APMA); Dr. Walter J. Pedowitz, M.D., associate clinical professor of orthopedic surgery, Columbia University; Wolfgang Brolley, physical therapist and licensed massage therapist; Susan Grote, physical therapist and yoga teacher; Dr. Emmanuel R. Loucas, M.D., dermatologist and fellow of the American Academy of Dermatology; Roger Marzano, C.P.O., C.Ped., past president of the Pedorthic Footwear Association.

My physical therapist, Shari Einhorn-Dicks, M.S.P.T., for taking care of my impossible feet.

Ted Johnson, M.D., and Vivian Lunny, M.D., and fellow of the International Federation of Aromatherapy, for their editorial suggestions.

Brad Crissman of the AOFAS, for his generous support during my research.

Debby Heath and Peter Cole for test-driving all of the stretches and exercises. Terence Pagard for his courier services.

Martha Buldain, reflexologist, for teaching me about essential oils, foot massage, and reflexology. Marcia Elston, herbalist and certified aromatherapist, for teaching me about essential oils and aromatherapy.

My mother, Joanne Dillman, for the countless foot-related newspaper and magazine clippings she sent me during my research.

My friends and family, for their support and encouragement.

Contents

CONTENTS

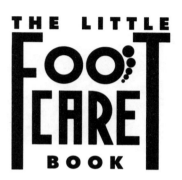

THE LITTLE FOOT CARE BOOK

1 Feet Don't Fail Me Now

*[The foot is] a masterpiece of engineering
and a work of art.*
—LEONARDO DA VINCI

Unfortunately, most of us don't think so highly of our feet. In fact, we don't think of them at all until they hurt.

The feet are one of the most abused and neglected parts of the body. They support our weight, they get crammed into high-heeled shoes, they take a pounding when we walk, dance, play sports, or stand on them all day long. They get hot, sweaty, itchy, and smelly. It's no wonder that 80 percent of Americans will have a foot problem in their lifetimes.[1]

So What Have You Done for Your Feet Lately?

Look around your bathroom, and you're likely to see several different hand lotions, shampoos, face creams, face scrubs, toners, cotton balls, and all the other products you use to keep your hands and face looking great. But what about your feet? They need attention, too.

In *The Little Foot Care Book* you'll learn how spending just a few minutes a day caring for your feet can help you feel good and prevent many common foot problems. It's true that if your feet feel good, you'll feel good. Your feet affect your balance, posture, and ability to be active. They contain thousands of nerve endings, and often your feet are indicators of overall health. Some illnesses, like arthritis, diabetes, or circulatory diseases, often first display symptoms in the feet.

Taking care of your feet is not difficult or time-consuming. In the amount of time it takes to apply hand lotion or wash your face, you can pamper your feet. *The Little Foot Care Book* is loaded with information on foot soaks, lotions, scrubs, massages, stretches, and more. Your feet will thank you for reading this book. After all, few things feel more luxurious than a soothing lavender foot soak or an invigorating peppermint foot massage at the end of a long day.

Foot Anatomy

The feet are complicated structures designed to support the body's weight and provide flexibility in movement. Each foot is an intricate network of 19 muscles, 26 bones (plus 2 sesamoid bones), 33 joints, and 107 ligaments, tendons, and nerves. The forefoot consists of 5 metatarsal bones, which bear most of the body's weight when walking, 2 sesamoid bones, and 14 phalanges (toe bones). The midfoot has 5 tarsal bones, which form the arch of the foot. The talus (ankle bone) and calcaneus (heel bone) form the hindfoot.

When you are standing, your body's weight is transferred through the ankle bone to the rest of the foot bones, with the hindfoot and midfoot absorbing most of the shock. Four arches in the foot also help carry and distribute weight: the transverse arch, the anterior metatarsal arch, the lateral arch, and the medial arch.

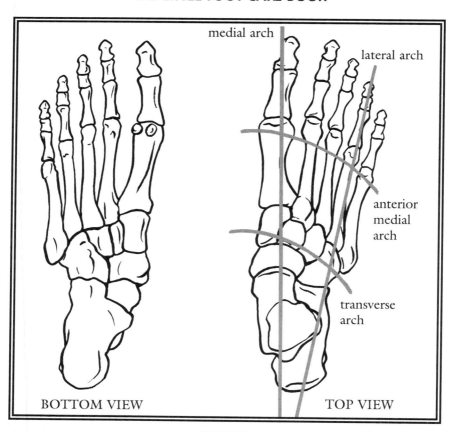

medial arch

lateral arch

anterior medial arch

transverse arch

BOTTOM VIEW

TOP VIEW

With such an elaborate structure, it's easy to see how even minor foot problems can throw your feet out of whack.

Foot Facts

- Twenty-five percent of the body's bones are in the feet.[2]
- Women have four times as many foot problems as men.[3]
- The average person takes 8,000–10,000 steps a day, and will walk more than 115,000 miles in a lifetime.[4]
- Two-thirds of Americans' 175 million foot problems are caused by improperly fitting shoes.[5]
- The average man walks seven miles a day; the average woman walks ten.[6]
- Each step you take produces a force of up to two times your body weight—three to four times your weight when running.[7]

HAPPY FEET CHECKLIST

Do you have happy feet? Do you:

1. Wash your feet every day?
2. Cut toenails straight across?
3. Exfoliate, soak, and moisturize your feet regularly?
4. Get a foot massage regularly (or give yourself one)?
5. Take care of small foot problems before they become big foot problems?
6. Wear socks made out of natural fibers, and change socks daily?
7. Wear comfortable, supportive shoes that fit the shape and size of your feet?
8. Wear shoes outside and during recreational activities (where going barefoot could put you at risk of cutting or injuring your feet)?
9. Avoid high heels?
10. Exercise: walk, stretch, strengthen?

How many of the checklist items are you already doing for your feet? Be kind to them, and they'll serve you for a lifetime.

2 Treat Your Feet

I cannot think clearly when my feet hurt.
—ABRAHAM LINCOLN

The best thing about foot pampering is that you don't need to go to a fancy spa or spend a lot of money to treat your feet; it's easy to do at home. In this chapter, you'll learn how to prepare soothing and relaxing foot soaks and how to make your own foot lotions, scrubs, and sprays using essential oils.

FOOT SOAKS

One of the simplest things you can do to treat your aching feet is soak them in a basin of warm water at the end of the day (or anytime you need relief). Foot soaks not only feel great; they can be very therapeutic. Soaking in warm water warms and re-laxes muscles, tendons, ligaments, and soft tissue, as well as in-creases circulation to the feet.

Cold soaks are also very beneficial to your feet because they increase circulation and reduce swelling. Cold soaks are best for inflammation or after strenuous activities like hiking, running, or other sports that might cause the feet to swell.

For maximum foot pampering, follow your foot soak with an exfoliating foot scrub and a self-massage with essential-oil foot lotion or cream (described later in this chapter.) **Health note:** Diabetics should not soak their feet. See page 186 for informa-tion on diabetic foot care.

Get Soaking

All you really need for a good foot soak is water and a basin, but there are a few ingredients that you'll want to have around the house so that you're always prepared to whip up a little basin of relaxation.

- Small pebbles or marbles. These can be added to the bottom of the basin. As you soak, you can rub your feet against them for a mini-massage.

- Bicarbonate of soda (baking soda). Good for soothing the feet and conditioning the skin.

- Epsom salt. Used in Chinese medicine to help draw toxins out of the feet, epsom salt soothes the skin and helps restore tired muscles. Dead Sea salt is full of minerals that are absorbed by your feet while they soak.

- Essential oils and herbs. These substances have a variety of medicinal properties (antiseptic, antibacterial, antifungal, anti-inflammatory) that can enhance a foot soak's therapeutic benefits, which might include: reducing inflammation; relieving painful, sore, aching, cramping muscles; softening and conditioning skin; and increasing circulation. While oils in a foot soak soothe your feet, their fragrance is also therapeutic and can be calming or stimulating, depending on which oils you use.

  The five oils you'll use most are lavender, peppermint,

rosemary, geranium, and tea tree. You might also like to have eucalyptus, cypress, sage, chamomile, and lemon. Use only therapeutic-grade oils. (See chart on pages 12–16.)

You might also want to keep these dried herbs around: peppermint, lavender, chamomile. And a few cotton muslin tea bags.

Essential Oils

Essential oils are highly concentrated natural substances extracted by steam distillation, or by other methods, from plant leaves, flowers, roots, and seeds. Throughout history, ancient cultures in Egypt, India, China, Rome, and Greece used aromatic oils for therapeutic and medicinal practices, in religious ceremonies, in cosmetic and perfume products, as well as for bathing.

Today the use of essential oils and the practice of aromatherapy are common around the world. There are two primary ways in which essential oils interact with the body: through inhalation or through absorption by the skin. Both methods can produce emotional and physical changes in the body. For example, lavender is widely known for its calming properties, even if it's simply inhaled. Peppermint is often used in massage to soothe aching limbs. Adding essential oils (and mineral salt) to a foot bath is doubly therapeutic because you can inhale the calming (or stimulating, depending on which oil is used) aroma of the oil, and at the same time your feet will absorb oil molecules and minerals from the salt. (Because warm water increases circulation in the feet, essential oils are absorbed better in warm soaks than in cold soaks.)

Aromatherapy is no simple science. Essential oils are complex structures with many beneficial, and even some harmful, properties. Always follow the instructions that come with the essential oils you buy, and always use therapeutic-grade oils sold by a knowledgeable dealer who can instruct you in their uses.

The ten essential oils listed below are commonly used substances that are easy to find in most herbal shops. I've listed only a few of the general properties and uses for each oil, concentrating mostly on uses related to foot care. For a more complete list of properties and uses, you might want to read an aromatherapy or essential oils book. If you want to use any of these oils for purposes other than those listed in the foot soaks, sprays, and potions sections of this book, consult your doctor and a certified aromatherapist to get a diagnosis and treatment plan for your specific condition.

Common Essential Oils	Properties and Uses
Cypress *(Cupresus sempervirens)*	Refreshing, deodorant. Used in massage oils/lotions and in foot soaks to soothe muscle cramps and rheumatism, relieve symptoms of menstrual and menopausal problems, and calm nervous tension. Also used for sweaty feet, and to treat some respiratory conditions.
Eucalyptus *(Eucalyptus globulus)*	Stimulating, decongestant, deodorant. Used in massage oils/lotions and in foot soaks to soothe arthritis, rheumatism, muscle aches and pains, and sprains. Also used to treat some skin problems and some respiratory conditions.

Common Essential Oils	Properties and Uses
Geranium *(Pelargonium graveolens)*	Stimulating, antidepressant. Used in massage oils/lotions and in foot soaks to reduce nervous tension, premenstrual syndrome (PMS), and other stress-related conditions. Increases circulation, good for dry skin.
Lavender *(Lavandula angustifolia)*	Calming, soothing, antidepressant. Used in massage oils/lotions and in foot soaks to soothe muscle aches and pains, cramps, sprains, and rheumatic conditions. Also used for many skin conditions, and for depression, insomnia, PMS, and nervous tension.
Lemon *(Citrus limon)*	Refreshing. Used in massage oils/lotions and in foot soaks to reduce anxiety and nervous tension, and as an astringent for the skin. *Warning: Lemon increases your risk of sunburn if left on skin. Wait six hours before exposing skin to sun, or cover skin where lotion was applied.*

Common Essential Oils	Properties and Uses
Peppermint *(Mentha piperita)*	Invigorating. Used in massage oils/lotions and in foot soaks to increase alertness, soothe muscle aches and pains, reduce inflammation, relieve headaches, and reduce fatigue. Also used for some skin conditions and to treat some respiratory conditions.
Roman chamomile *(Anthemis nobilis)*	Calming. Used in massage oils/lotions, and in foot soaks, to reduce anxiety, PMS, insomnia, nervous tension, and stress headaches. Also used in lotion for dry skin.
Rosemary *(Rosmarinus officinalis)*	Stimulating. Used in massage oils/lotions and in foot soaks to increase circulation; reduce painful, aching joints and gout; soothe muscle pain; relieve headaches, mental fatigue, nervous exhaustion, and stress. Also used to treat some respiratory and skin problems.

Common Essential Oils	Properties and Uses
Sage (*Salvia officinalis*)	Astringent, anti-inflammatory, antiseptic, antifungal. Used in massage oils/lotions and in foot soaks to relieve pain from arthritis, rheumatism, and sprains. Also used to treat sweaty, smelly feet. *Warning: Sage is a powerful substance that, if overused, could be harmful. Use with care; don't use more than three times a week.*
Tea tree (*Melaleuca alternifolia*)	Anti-inflammatory, antiseptic, and antifungal. Used in massage oils/lotions and in foot soaks to treat a variety of skin conditions, including bacterial and fungal infections (athlete's foot), viral infections (warts), and smelly feet. Also used to treat some respiratory conditions.

Common Essential Oils	Properties and Uses
Carrier oils	Just a few drops of an essential oil go a long way. They should always be diluted in a carrier oil, or, in the case of foot baths, in water. A few of the common carrier oils are: sweet almond oil, grapeseed oil, sunflower oil, olive oil, and jojoba oil. (See page 35 for more information about carrier oils.)

Dilutions

A general rule is 1–4 drops of essential oil per tablespoon of carrier oil (or lotion). It's always best to start with a few drops, adding one drop at a time. More equals better does not apply here. Here are a few general dilution guidelines for different products:

Soaks	5–6 drops in basin containing 2 or more gallons of water
Lotions	5–6 drops per ounce of lotion

Scrubs   5–6 drops per ounce of carrier oil

Sprays   5–6 drops per ounce of water

Health Notes:

- If you are pregnant, taking prescription medications (or herbs or homeopathic remedies), or have diabetes, epilepsy, heart disease or high blood pressure, or other medical conditions, consult with your doctor before using essential oils or any of the recipes in this book. You should also talk to a certified aromatherapist, who can tell you which essential oils might aggravate (or benefit) your specific health problem.

- Some people are very sensitive to these substances, so if you develop a skin rash or have any unpleasant reactions to the oils, see your doctor.

Safety, Storage, and Mixing Tips

- Essential oils should not be used undiluted on the skin. Always dilute essential oils in a carrier oil. It is safe to add a few drops of essential oil to a foot spritzer or foot bath because the water serves as a carrier. In some cases, lavender oil and tea tree oil can be applied directly to the skin in very small amounts (do not apply both oils at the same time).

- Never use essential oils internally, near the eyes, or on mucous membranes (i.e., inside mouth or nose). Follow the instructions and warnings that come with the oils. Keep out of children's reach. Do not use essential oils on children unless directed by your physician.

- Skin-test oils by diluting a small amount and applying it to the skin. If your skin becomes red or itchy, do not use that oil.

- Essential oils should be stored in dark-colored glass bottles. Make sure that the bottles are sealed tightly and stored in a cool, dark place (a wooden cabinet is ideal).

- For best results, use only therapeutic-grade oils distributed by reputable companies. Read up on essential oils before using them, and ask a certified aromatherapist for some basic instructions. If you prefer not to invest in several bottles of oil, you can ask your aromatherapist to mix the potions for you.

- When mixing oils, use essential oils sparingly. You will gain therapeutic benefits from just a few drops. It's best to start off with one or two drops, adding one drop at a time so that you can test the mixture. Essential oils are very strong; a little goes a long way.

Fancy Foot Soaks

Here are ten types of foot soaks developed to address all sorts of foot woes. Mix these soaks slowly, adding oils one drop at a time. If you are sensitive to aromas, you may want to alter the recipes and use fewer drops of essential oils. You might also want to spend some time sampling different oils at an herbal shop before you buy them so that you can pick the aromas that you think you will enjoy the most.

All of these soak recipes, as well as the lotions and sprays in this chapter, have been reviewed and approved by two certified aromatherapists, one who is also an M.D.

Tips:
- Place the basin on a thick towel to keep it warm and to catch any spills. You can also cover your feet and the basin with another towel to trap in the heat from the water (try to keep the top towel from touching the water).

- If you do add a few handfuls of marbles to your bath, make sure that the marbles are all smooth and don't have any chips that could cut your feet. You can also add river rocks or small smooth pebbles, which can be found at nurseries, gardening shops, craft shops, and stores that sell fountain supplies.

- For a good presoak foot massage and to exfoliate dry skin, fill another basin with sand. Sitting or standing, you can massage your feet into the sand.

Basic Soak

Here's a basic soak recipe to get you started:

1. Add warm water (not hot) to a basin or small tub until it's about two-thirds full.

2. Add 2 tbsp of either baking soda or salt to the water. Your measurements don't have to be exact; pour 1 tbsp into your palm so that you can see how much it holds, then you can just add 1–3 palmfuls. Don't use too much salt because it can be dehydrating. (In any of the recipes in this chapter, feel free to substitute epsom salt for mineral or Dead Sea salt; it's much cheaper.)

3. Add 3–5 drops of therapeutic-grade essential oil or 1–2 tbsp of herbs in a muslin tea bag. Stir water gently to disperse oil and dissolve salt.

4. Soak for 15–20 minutes.

De-Stress Soaks

After a long day, you need to calm your nerves and relax your mind. These "after-work" soaks are simple to make, using ingredients you might have in your kitchen.

Simple soak: Add 2 tbsp baking soda or epsom salt to a basin of warm water. Soak for 15–20 minutes.

Lavender soak: Add 2 tbsp baking soda and 5 drops of lavender oil to a basin of warm water. Soak for 15–20 minutes.

Zippy citrus soak: Add a few slices of lemon (or orange) and a few slices of fresh ginger to warm water. Squeeze the juice of a few slices into the water. Soak for 15–20 minutes. You can add 2 tbsp baking soda or salt to this soak. You can also substitute 3–5 drops of lemon oil for the slices.

REJUVENATING SOAKS

When you have time for a breather, but you need to keep going, a reenergizing soak will get you back on your feet.

Simple soak: Soak your feet in a basin of cold water for 15–20 minutes. You can add one or two trays of ice to make it colder. You can also add 3–5 drops of eucalyptus or peppermint oil.

Vitamin soak: Crush 2,000 mg of vitamin C (or use powdered vitamin C) into warm or cold water. Add 2 drops of eucalyptus oil, 2 drops of lavender oil, and 2 drops of rosemary oil. Soak for 15–20 minutes.

Peppy midday tea soak: Add 2 tbsp Dead Sea salt and 1 tbsp dried peppermint in a muslin tea bag (or use 3–5 drops of peppermint oil) to a basin of warm water. Soak for 15–20 minutes.

THERAPEUTIC SOAKS

Whether you have arthritis, gout, or rheumatism, or stiff, inflamed, and sore joints from overuse, this soak will cool down your feet and increase circulation. If your feet feel painful and hot, do a cold soak. If your feet feet achy and tired, do a warm soak. (See page 141 for information on arthritis.)

Rosemary soak: Add 2 tbsp Dead Sea salt (or baking soda), 3–5 drops of rosemary oil, and 2 trays of ice to a basin of cold water. (For warm soak, add ingredients to a basin of warm water. Do not add ice.) Soak for 15–20 minutes.

Sore joints soak: Add 2 drops of eucalyptus oil, 2 drops of rosemary oil, and 1 drop of lavender oil to a basin of cold water. Add 2 trays of ice cubes. (For warm soak, add ingredients to a basin of warm water. Do not add ice.) Soak for 15–20 minutes.

If you have cramps or stiffness in your feet, try these soothing soaks, which are also good for sweaty feet and for calming your nerves:

Stiff feet soak 1: Add 3 drops of cypress oil and 3 drops of lemon oil to a basin of warm water. You can also add 2 tbsp of epsom salt. Soak for 15–20 minutes.

Stiff feet soak 2: Add 3 drops of rosemary oil and 3 drops of lavender oil to a basin of warm water. You can also add 2 tbsp of epsom salt. Soak for 15–20 minutes.

Bunion soak: Add 2 tbsp epsom salt, 2 tbsp olive (or safflower) oil, 3 drops of eucalyptus oil, 1 drop of sage oil, and 1 drop of rosemary oil to a basin of warm water. Soak for 15–20 minutes.

BEDTIME SOAKS

An hour before bedtime is a perfect time to do a foot soak that will help you relax and fall asleep.

Oatmeal soak: Add ¼–½ cup dried oats (i.e., oatmeal, but don't use instant) to a basin of warm water. You can also add 3–5 drops of lavender oil or throw in a few bags of chamomile tea (decaffeinated!). Soak for 15–20 minutes.

Sleepy soak: Add 2 tbsp dried lavender in a muslin tea bag and 2 tbsp epsom salt to a basin of warm water. Soak 15–20 minutes. (Although dried herbs take a few more minutes to use, they are perfect for bedtime teas since they're a bit less fragrant than oils. Some people who are extremely sensitive to fragrance can be overstimulated by strong scents, so they should use dried herbs before bed.)

RELAXING SOAKS

When you want to unwind, unplug from the chaos, and feel a little pampered, try this soak:

Soothing soak: Add 3 drops of chamomile oil, 2 drops of lavender oil, and 2–3 tbsp Dead Sea salt to a basin of warm water. Soak for 15–20 minutes.

When PMS strikes and you begin to feel depressed, irritable, bloated, and fatigued, put your feet up for a few minutes and rest. Then, take a soak:

PMS soak: Add 3 tbsp Dead Sea salt and 3–5 drops of geranium oil to a basin of warm water. Soak for 15–20 minutes. Afterward, give yourself a foot massage with lavender foot lotion (see page 53).

For those days when everyone is getting on your last nerve, lock yourself in your house and soak away.

Foot soak for cranks: Add 2 tbsp epsom salt, 2 drops of peppermint oil, 3 drops of rosemary oil, and 1 drop of lavender oil to a basin of warm water. Soak for 15–20 minutes.

AFTER-WORKOUT SOAKS

Your dogs are barkin'! You just hiked ten miles, and you need to bring some life back into your tired, overworked, swollen, smelly feet. If your feet are painful, bruised, or swollen, first soak in cold, icy water for 20 minutes. Wait 30–60 minutes, and then do one of these warm soaks:

Hiker's soak: Add 2–3 tbsp Dead Sea salt (or epsom salt), 1 drop of tea tree oil, 2 drops of lavender oil, and 2 drops of rosemary oil to a basin of warm water. Soak for 15–20 minutes.

Runner's soak: Add 2 tbsp epsom salts and 1 pinch (⅛–¼ tsp) of cayenne pepper to a basin of warm water. Soak for 15–20 minutes.

Sore feet soak: Add 2 tbsp mineral or Dead Sea salt, 2 drops of lavender oil, and 3 drops of eucalyptus oil to a basin of warm water. Soak for 15–20 minutes.

"MY FEET ARE KILLING ME" SOAKS

When your feet are tired, aching, swollen, and you just can't go on . . .

Basic soak: Add 2 tbsp baking soda, 3 drops of cypress oil, and 3 drops of lavender oil to a basin of warm water. Soak for 15–20 minutes.

Fancy soak: Add 2 tbsp Dead Sea salt, 2 drops of eucalyptus oil, 2 drops of peppermint oil, 1 drop of lavender oil, and 1 drop of rosemary oil to a basin of warm water. Soak for 15–20 minutes.

STINKY FEET SOAKS

First, try a soak to combat sweaty feet. Then try the recipes for smelly feet. (See page 178 for information on smelly feet.)

Sweaty feet soak: Add 3 drops of cypress oil and 2 drops of sage oil (optional) to a basin of warm water. Squeeze several slices of lemon into the water, and add the slices (or add 1 drop of lemon oil). Soak for 15–20 minutes.

Odor-eater tea: Make a pint of tea, using 2 tea bags. Boil for 15 minutes (with tea bags in the water). Add tea to 2 quarts of cool water, and soak in the cool solution for 30 minutes. Black tea contains tannic acid, which kills bacteria and closes pores, so soaking feet in strong black tea for 30 minutes a day for a week can sometimes help keep your feet dryer during the day.

Pickled feet soak: You can also soak your feet in vinegar. Make a solution of one part vinegar to two parts water in your basin and soak for 20 minutes. Use room-temperature water; warm water can increase the vinegar fumes.

Tea tree soak: Add 2 tbsp baking soda, 3 drops of tea tree oil, 1 drop of geranium oil, and 2 drops of lavender oil to a basin of warm water. Soak for 20 minutes.

HEADACHE SOAK

A warm herbal foot bath can help you relax and unwind, which is sometimes all you need to alleviate some headaches. Breathing deeply while you soak will also help calm your mind, as you inhale the aromatic oil in the bath. Sometimes a calming oil works best, sometimes a stimulating oil works best, and sometimes it takes a combination of oils. Experiment and see which oils work for you.

Headache soak: Add 3–5 drops of one of the following oils to a basin of warm water: lavender (calming), peppermint (stimulating), eucalyptus (stimulating and great for congestion), or rosemary (stimulating, rejuvenating). Soak for 15–20 minutes.

POTIONS & LOTIONS, SCRUBS, AND SPRAYS

In addition to soaking your feet, taking care of the skin on your feet is the next step in foot pampering. For a complete foot treatment, you'll want to exfoliate (scrub away dead skin cells on) the bottoms of your feet after soaking, pat them dry, and apply a moisturizer. You can buy a variety of moisturizing lotions, exfoliating scrubs, and refreshing sprays for your feet, or you can make them at home with a few easy-to-find ingredients.

Using essential oils, Dead Sea salt, a carrier oil, and fragrance-free lotion, you can make your own foot scrubs, aromatherapy lotions and oils, and foot sprays. You'll want to buy several 1-, 2-, and 4-ounce containers in which to store your potions.

Fancy Foot Scrub

Place one cup of chunky mineral salt in a bowl. Drizzle a teaspoon of carrier oil over the salt so that the surface of the salt is covered with a thin layer of oil. Add 5 drops of essential oil (lavender, peppermint, or eucalyptus). Gently mix together oils and salt. Store in plastic or glass container. The essential oil will stay potent for six months.

After your foot soak, scrub your foot with a handful of salt, rubbing the salt into your feet using a circular motion. Pay extra attention to the areas of your feet that have dry, hard skin. Rinse well. Pat dry with a towel and apply moisturizing lotion or cream.

Fancy Foot Lotion

The simplest way to benefit from essential oils is to add several drops of your favorite oil to a bottle of fragrance-free moisturizing lotion or cream. (Products that are marked "unscented" often have masking agents in them to hide the scent, so look for the words "fragrance-free.") Because the skin on the bottom of your feet is usually drier than anywhere else on your body, you might prefer to use cream instead of lotion because it can be more effective at sealing moisture into the skin. (See page 166 for more information on dry skin.)

Buy the purest product you can find, one that has the fewest preservatives and chemicals. Lubriderm, Eucerin, and Amlactin are all good lotions easily found at supermarkets and drugstores. You can also order lotions from suppliers listed in the back of the book or buy them at your local natural foods market or herbal shop. Instead of adding essential oils directly into your lotion, buy several 1-ounce containers so that you can make a variety of scented lotions.

Add 3–5 drops of essential oil per ounce of lotion. Rub lotion into your feet, kneading your arches and massaging your ankles and toes. If you like strongly scented lotions, you can add 1–2 more drops of essential oil to your lotion.

Here are some of my favorite lotions with quantities given for a 1-oz. bottle:

1. 5 drops of lavender + lotion
2. 2 drops of peppermint + 2 drops of rosemary + 1 drop of lavender + lotion
3. 5 drops of peppermint + lotion
4. 2 drops of lemon + 3 drop of eucalyptus + lotion

Fancy Foot Oil

You can make your own massage oil very easily by adding a few drops of your favorite essential oils to a carrier oil.

The most inexpensive carrier oils to use you probably already have in your house: olive oil, safflower oil, sunflower oil, or basic vegetable oil. You can also buy carrier oils at massage supply stores, natural food markets, and even at many supermarkets. Sweet almond oil is ideal, but don't forget to store it, or any carrier oils, in the refrigerator to preserve freshness. Both sweet almond oil and jojoba oil (which is actually a wax) are easy to find at natural food markets, herbal stores, and massage suppliers.

Sweet almond, sunflower, and safflower oils can all be used at 100 percent strength, but if you use olive oil or jojoba oil, use them in 10 percent dilution (i.e., only 10 percent of the mixture should contain olive or jojoba oil). Also, olive oil can have a strong smell, so it's good to use it as part of a blend with another oil.

The basic rule of thumb for blending is 5 drops of essential oil for each ounce of carrier oil. For a 4-ounce bottle, that's 20–24 drops.

Fancy Foot Sprays

When you don't have the time or the room for a foot soak, foot sprays can revive your feet, rejuvenate your spirit, and even protect you from locker room germs. These sprays feel refreshing on your skin, but don't leave it greasy like some lotions can.

What you need to get started

- A few 4- and 2-ounce spray bottles (plastic containers are best for traveling and locker room use). Most of these recipes are based on 4-ounce containers; you can pour mixtures into two 2-ounce containers for travel-size sprays.

- You can make these recipes yourself or, if you don't want to invest in all of the different essential oils, pick a few recipes that look good to you and have an aromatherapist make them up for you.

- Use distilled water.

Tips:
- Let new sprays sit for a few days before you use them.

- The essential oils in the sprays will remain potent for six months. Shake well before use to disperse oils. Store in a cool, dark place.

- If you want a more moisturizing spray, you can add 1 tbsp of carrier oil to the water before adding the essential oils. You can also add an emulsifier to the mixture to help disperse the oils. Contact one of the herbal/essential oil suppliers listed in the back of the book for more information on emulsifiers.

Health note: Do not use essential oils if you have epilepsy or any of the other conditions listed starting on page 141.

GYM BAG SPRAY

Who knows what kind of fungus, germs, and bacteria are lurking on the floors of your health club locker room? Here's a spray that will refresh your feet after working out, and at the same time combat the creepy crawlies. (See page 146 for information on athlete's foot.)

Pour distilled water into a 4-ounce spray bottle, but don't fill it all the way to the top. Add the following essential oils, in the order listed:

6 drops of lavender oil
3 drops of tea tree oil
4 drops of peppermint oil
7 drops of lemon oil

Fill the rest of the bottle with distilled water. Shake before using to disperse oils.

SMELLY FOOT SPRAY

If your feet pour on the sweat when you exercise, here's a spray to keep them smelling nice. Use before working out. Spray on feet, on socks, and in shoes.

Pour distilled water into a 4-ounce spray bottle, but don't fill it all the way to the top. Add the following essential oils, in the order listed:

8 drops of cypress oil
2 drops of sage oil
3 drops of eucalyptus oil
1 drop of lemon oil

Fill the rest of the bottle with distilled water. Shake before using to disperse oils.

Health note: Sage should be used with caution; too much sage can be harmful. Use this spray only three times a week.

Use smaller, 2-ounce bottles for the rest of the soaks in this chapter so that you can take them with you wherever you go.

You can also double the recipes if you prefer using 4-ounce bottles.

REVIVING FOOT SPRAY

When your feet need a little refreshment, spray them with this tonic.

Backpacker's spray: Pour distilled water into a 2-ounce spray bottle, but don't fill it all the way to the top. Add the following essential oils, in the order listed:

5 drops of peppermint oil
4 drops of rosemary oil
3 drops of lavender oil

Fill the rest of the bottle with distilled water. Shake before using to disperse oils.

Everyday spray: Pour distilled water into a 2-ounce bottle, but don't fill it all·the way to the top. Add the following essential oils, in the order listed:

5 drops of peppermint oil
4 drops of rosemary oil
1 drop of tea tree oil
1 drop of geranium oil

Fill the rest of the bottle with distilled water. Shake before using to disperse oils.

INVIGORATING FOOT SPRAYS

Pick-me-up spray: Pour distilled water into a 2-ounce spray bottle, but don't fill it all the way to the top. Add the following essential oils, in the order listed:

2 drops of tea tree oil
4 drops of eucalyptus oil
3 drops of rosemary oil
1 drop of lemon oil

Fill the rest of the bottle with distilled water. Shake before using to disperse oils.

Zesty lemon spray: Pour distilled water into a 2-ounce spray bottle, but don't fill it all the way to the top. Add the following essential oil:

5 drops of lemon oil

Fill the rest of the bottle with distilled water. Shake before using to disperse oil.

3 Spa Feet

Put your best foot forward.
—ROBERT BROWNING

Anyone who's ever had a great pedicure knows that there are few things that rival the bliss of having so much attention lavished on your feet.

Professional Pedicures

Most day spas and salons offer pedicures; for $35–$65 you get a one-hour treatment that will leave you feeling relaxed and rejuvenated. Professional pedicures generally include a cleansing foot soak; filing of corns, calluses, and dry skin areas; a moisturizing treatment; cuticle shaping; nail trimming and cleaning; and the application of nail polish. Some pedicures also include a brief foot massage.

If you do go to a salon for your pedicure, make sure that the pedicurist is experienced, licensed, and working at a reputable spa or salon. Your pedicurist should have her state license posted at her work station. When you call for an appointment, you can ask about qualifications, training, and licensing.

Health note: There are a few things that professional pedicurists should not do to your feet, especially if you have diabetes. If you need your corns and calluses shaved or cut, or if you need your cuticles cut, see a doctor.

Sterilization

The most important question to ask when you call for a pedicure appointment is what procedure the salon has in place to properly sterilize the pedicure implements. Procedures may differ from state to state and from salon to salon. Some pedicurists scrub used implements with a brush and soap, then soak them in disinfectant solution for 20–30 minutes. Some also place implements in steam or dry heat. Implements should be stored in sterile containers. Find out if the salon's procedures include some form of sterilization using hospital-grade disinfectant solution that kills bacteria, fungus, and viruses like HIV and hepatitis. Some salons may use disposable implements, or include in the cost of the pedicure your own kit that you can bring with you each time you have a pedicure.

Some implements, like emery boards and orange sticks, cannot be cleaned and should be thrown away after use.

Home Pedicures

If you don't have the time, money, or energy to get a professional pedicure, give yourself one at home. Better yet, invite a friend over and give each other pedicures.

Pedicure Products

Many cosmetic companies now have special foot care lines, so it shouldn't be hard to find plenty of products for your home pedicure. Most drugstores and grocery stores sell inexpensive pedicure kits that include orange sticks, foam toe separators, and files, as well as a variety of scrubs, soaks, and lotions. Dr. Scholl's makes a complete pedicure line, and the products are easy to find and reasonably priced. You can also find pedicure products at salons, spas, and bath shops.

If you're going to invest in a few top-of-the-line products, buy a good foot file and good oil or lotion for your nails. Diamancel diamond foot files are ideal for pedicures and are used at some of the best spas and salons. These strong, durable files last forever and can be safety cleaned and soaked in antibacterial solution. Dr. Hauschka's Neem Oil for Nails, which contains Indian neem oil, chamomile extract, and lavender oil, is a great treatment for softening cuticles and preventing nails from cracking. For foot soaks, try Dr. Singha's Mustard Bath or EO's peppermint and lavender foot salts.

What you'll need

- Basin of warm water (with mild soap, bath salts, and/or essential oils)
- File or pumice stone
- Toenail clippers and orange stick (a thin wooden stick with one beveled edge)
- Foam toe separator (or cotton balls) and polish
- Lotion and towels

Instructions

1. Soak your feet in warm water to soften and clean the skin. (See page 19 for soak recipes.)

2. Pat your feet dry with a towel (wiping or rubbing your feet dry with a towel absorbs too much moisture), making sure that you dry between your toes.

3. Exfoliate, which means get rid of dead skin cells on the surface of your feet. Using a pumice stone, gently scrub your corns, calluses, and the dry skin on your heels, toes,

and along the edges of your feet with back-and-forth movements. You may want to wet the stone first. Don't scrub too hard or too deep because you can burn your skin. It's better to remove dead skin in many small increments over a period of time.

If you would rather use a file, the procedure is slightly different. Filing is most effective when done on dry feet, so if you use a file instead of a pumice stone, file your feet before you soak. (Read the instructions that come with your file or pumice stone. Some pedicurists recommend exfoliating dry feet, and some podiatrists recommend exfoliating wet feet. Likewise, some implements work better on dry feet or on wet feet.) Do not try to cut off your corns or calluses; leave that to a doctor who has the proper equipment and experience. As with the pumice stone, be very gentle as you file, and file your feet in small increments to prevent damaging your skin. Do yourself a favor and invest in a good file.

You can also use an exfoliating salt scrub, which you can make yourself (see page 32) or buy at the store.

4. Massage a little dab of lotion or oil into your cuticles to soften them. Beginning at one end of your nail and moving across the nail to the other side, gently push back your cuticles using an orange stick with a little bit of cotton from a cotton ball wrapped around the tip to protect your skin from the sharp edge. Repeat for each of your toes. When you are finished, make sure that you wipe all of the lotion or oil off your nails. Do not cut your cuticles because they protect the nail bed from infection. If you think your cuticles need trimming, see your podiatrist.

5. Clean under your nails with a softened orange stick. To soften it, soak it in water for a few minutes or wrap a piece of cotton around the tip. Metal implements should not be used to clean under your nails because they can tear the tissue under your nail, increasing your risk of infection.

6. Cut your toenails with toenail clippers, making sure that you cut your nails straight across to prevent ingrown toenails. It will be easier to cut your nails with a straight edge if you use several small clips to slowly work your way across each nail instead of trying to clip an entire nail in

one cut. Toenails should be dry when you cut them, and don't cut your nails too short. You can file the edges of your toenails with an emery board or file (use a much finer-surfaced file for filing nails than the one you used for filing calluses). Be careful not to cut too deeply into the groove between the big toenail and the skin surrounding it.

7. Moisturize your feet with foot cream or lotion, massaging your feet as you apply the lotion. You can make your own foot lotion (see page 33), or buy your favorite lotion at the store. Your pedicure can end after this step, or if you want to paint your nails, follow the next four steps.

8. Before you apply any nail polish, you'll need to remove all of the lotion from your toenails. You can wash them with soapy water or give them a swipe with a cotton ball that has a few drops of rubbing alcohol on it.

9. Separate your toes with a foam toe separator or with cotton balls. Apply nail polish one toe at a time, painting from the base of the nail to the top of the nail. Allow

about 5 minutes for the base coat to dry (less time if you are using quick-drying polish). Then apply one or two coats of whatever color polish you like, allowing time between coats for drying. Finally, apply a clear top coat to protect the color from chipping. Wait about 15–20 minutes for nails to dry completely before putting on your socks and shoes.

10. If you are the only person using your pedicure implements, and you don't have any foot infections, you can save your orange sticks and emery boards. Otherwise, throw them away after use. You can scrub your metal implements with a small brush and soap, then soak them in an antibacterial solution. If you're the only one using them, spraying or wiping them with Lysol, peroxide, or alcohol should provide adequate cleaning. You can clean the basin you soak in with these products, too.

11. You can give yourself a pedicure every few weeks, especially during the spring and summer months, when your feet will be on display in sandals. If you're getting salon pedicures, it's good to go for a polish change every three

to four weeks. Occasionally, you might also want to go without polish for a few weeks between pedicures to give your toenails some air.

Health notes: If you have diabetes or circulatory problems, consult your doctor before getting a pedicure.

If your doctor has diagnosed you with toenail fungus, do not paint your toenails until they heal because the polish can trap moisture and infection in the nails. (See page 175 for more information about toenail fungus.)

4 Rub Some Life into Your Feet

Make your foot your friend.
—J. M. BARRIE

FOOT MASSAGE

Few things feel more soothing than a good foot massage. With more than 70,000 nerve endings in your feet, it's no wonder that reducing tension and fatigue in your feet promotes relaxation and revitalization throughout your entire body.

Your feet deserve some attention. Most people throw on their socks and shoes every morning without ever thinking about their feet. Just holding your feet between your hands or soaking them in a warm foot bath is a great way to start getting in touch with your feet. When you become more aware of what your feet need to feel good, you'll want to include some foot pampering in your daily routine.

Massage relaxes the muscles and tissues of the feet, increases circulation in the feet, helps the body eliminate toxins, reduces tension, and promotes relaxation.

Self-Massage

One of the best things about foot massage is that, unlike your back and shoulders, your feet are easy to reach with both hands so you don't have to wait for an appointment with a massage therapist; you can work on your own feet whenever you want. With a few simple strokes you can bring your feet back to life.

- First, warm and wash your feet with a 10- to 15-minute foot soak. (See soaks on pages 7–31.) After your soak, pat your feet dry with a towel, making sure to dry between the toes.

- You can use a little bit of oil or lotion (a drop about the size of a dime) to massage your feet, but don't use too much, or your feet will be too slippery. Adding essential oils to your carrier oil or unscented lotion is another way to increase the benefits of your foot massage, since the soles of the feet will absorb the essential oils. For revitalizing tired, aching feet, use peppermint oil, which feels tingly and refreshing against the skin. Eucalyptus oil also feels very cool against the skin but at the same time warms the muscles. See page 33 for instructions on how to make therapeutic massage lotions and oils.

ORDER OF TREATMENT

The foot massage below can be a complete treatment in itself, or for maximum pampering you can follow your massage with a few reflexology techniques, which are described on pages 67–68.

INSTRUCTIONS

1. Sitting in a comfortable, supportive chair or couch, or on the floor, place the outside ankle of your left foot on your right thigh.

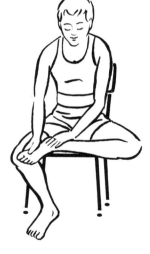

2. Rub a drop of oil or lotion between your hands to warm it up, then gently stroke and rub your foot until it's covered with the oil or lotion.

3. Support your left foot by holding it with your left hand and begin to stroke the bottom of your foot with the knuckles of your right hand from your heels to your toes. Then, starting at the bottom of your heel and working your way up to the base of your toes, press your knuckles into the bottom of your foot. Move your knuckles up the foot by rolling them side to side while applying pressure. (Relaxing the toes will help keep the bottom of the foot relaxed and pliable.)

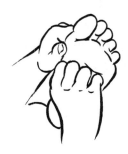

4. Still supporting your left foot, massage each of your toes. Start at the base of your big toe, squeezing between the joints of the toe. Then repeat the same for each of your toes, ending with your little toe.

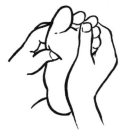

5. Beginning with the big toe again, roll your toe between your fingers as you gently pull it away from the foot. Repeat for all of your toes, ending with your little toe.

6. Holding the outside of your left foot with your right hand, grasp your toes with your left hand and slowly move them forward and backward to give them a good stretch.

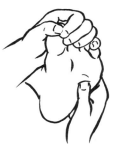

7. Hold your left foot in both hands, with thumbs pressed against sole of foot, one thumb over the other. Press thumbs firmly into sole of foot and slide your thumbs up to the ball of your foot. Keep applying pressure as you slide thumbs away from each other across the ball of foot. Repeat a few times.

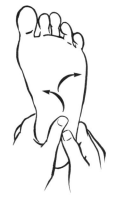

8. Change your position so that you're sitting with your left leg bent, left foot placed against the edge of the couch (or flat against the floor if you're sitting on the floor). Get another small dab of oil or lotion and rub it between your hands. Rub the oil into your lower leg from your calf to your ankle.

9. Hold on to your left calf so that your fingers are wrapped around the front of your lower leg and your thumbs are crossed, one on top of the other, at your calf muscles. Applying pressure with your thumbs, slide down the back of your leg. Repeat, moving your thumbs slightly to the left and slide down the back of your leg again. Do the same on your right side. Repeat sequence a few times. Then massage around your ankle. You can rest your left foot on your thigh again and rotate your foot several times, first clockwise, then counterclockwise. Then make circles around your ankle using your thumbs (or your fingers). You can massage your ankle sitting or in the same position as you used in massaging your calf.

10. Repeat steps 1 through 9 on your right foot.

Tip: Some people who have repetitive strain injury or carpal tunnel problems in their arms and wrists may find foot massage and reflexology difficult to do. If you can't use your hands, fingers, or thumbs, try using some of the massage and reflexology tools on pages 77–80 to give yourself a massage.

A LITTLE BIT OF REFLEXOLOGY

What Is Reflexology?

Reflexology is a type of foot massage in which pressure is applied to points on the feet to stimulate balance, well-being, and healing throughout the body.

Reflexology is based on the principle that there are ten energy zones in the body (running from head to toes, similar to the meridians on which acupuncture is based) and points on the feet (called reflex points) that correspond to specific body parts. The goal of a reflexology treatment is to restore the body's natural balance by eliminating or reducing conditions like inflammation, congestion, and physical or emotional tension that block energy in the body.

Treating the whole body through the feet is nothing new. Holistic foot massage therapies were commonly used in China 5,000 years ago, and paintings and hieroglyphics found on the walls of Egyptian tombs have illustrated that reflex treatments were practiced in Egypt more than 4,000 years ago. Other countries, like India and Japan, have their own healing traditions of reflexology. In this country, Native Americans in the

1700s used foot reflex treatments in their healing practices. You just need to look on the bookshelves in the health section of most bookstores to see that reflexology has become a well-known and respected treatment in this country and throughout the world.

How Does Reflexology Work?

Reflexology is based on the belief that the entire body is represented in the feet. One of the most important benefits of reflexology is relaxation. By reflexing points on the feet that correspond to specific body parts or organs, a reflexology treatment can reduce stress and tension, which in turn frees up the body's energy for healing or simply facing the stresses of everyday life.

The following chart describes the reflex points and their corresponding body areas:

Toes	Head and neck: eyes, sinuses, brain.
Ball of foot	Chest, lungs, shoulders.
Arch	Stomach, pancreas, adrenals, kidney, spleen, solar plexus, gallbladder, liver, colon.
Heel	Sciatic nerve, pelvis: bladder, rectum.
Outside edge of foot	Arms and legs.
Inside edge of foot	Spine.
Ankle	Pelvis: ovaries/testes, uterus/prostate, rectum.

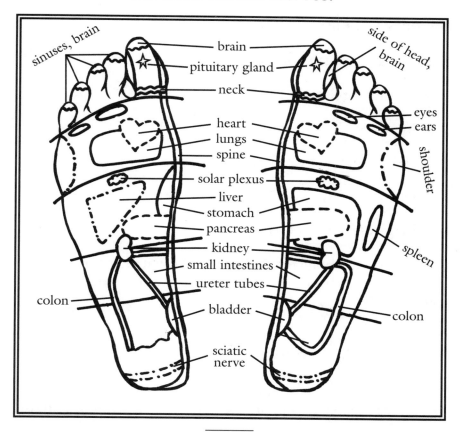

sinuses, brain

side of head, brain

brain

pituitary gland

neck

eyes

ears

heart

lungs

spine

shoulder

solar plexus

liver

stomach

pancreas

spleen

kidney

small intestines

ureter tubes

colon

bladder

colon

sciatic
nerve

Benefits of Reflexology

Reflexology has many of the same benefits as massage; it

- Promotes relaxation

- Improves circulation

- Helps eliminate toxins in the body

- Balances body and mind

- Reduces stress and tension

The best thing about reflexology is that, whether you feel the referral benefits or not, it feels great to have someone work on your feet.

Finding a Reflexologist

Most spas and massage centers offer reflexology, in addition to the many reflexologists in private practice. A good reflexologist should be trained and certified by a reputable massage or re-flexology school. Reflexology sessions last anywhere from half an hour to an hour and a half. Expect to pay $20–$35 for a half-hour session, $40–$70 for an hour session, and $80–$95 for an hour and a half session. For a budget massage or reflexology treatment, contact the massage schools in your area. Schools often offer free or discounted treatments to people willing to be part of a student training session.

Self-Reflexology

You can also give yourself reflexology. The illustrations and maps may look confusing, but don't let them intimidate you. Just pressing on the different areas of the foot with your thumbs and fingers can be surprisingly calming and effective.

Here are a few general guidelines to keep in mind:

1. Sit in a comfortable and supportive chair so that you can easily rest the foot on which you will be working across the thigh of your other leg. If this position isn't comfortable, you

can sit on the floor or find another position that is comfortable.

2. Reflexology can be done on a dry foot or with a small amount of lotion. You want to have a little bit of friction between your fingers and the skin of your foot. Be careful not to use too much lotion. If the surface of your foot is too slippery, you won't be able to properly reflex the foot points.

3. Don't worry about getting the technique perfect; your goal is simply to pamper your feet, not pass a reflexology training course. There are many, many different styles and techniques used in reflexology. This book includes just a sampling of techniques to get you started. If you reflex the different areas of your feet, you will gain benefits. Also, don't feel bad about altering some of the directions to suit your needs. For example, if the instructions tell you to walk up the toe and it's easier for you to get your hand and foot in a position to walk down the toe, do what's most comfortable for your body.

4. If any of the massage or reflexology techniques you try make your feet or hands uncomfortable or painful, stop the ses-

sion. Sometimes changing positions might make it more comfortable for you. If the pain continues, it could be a sign of an underlying strain or injury, and you should consult your doctor and a reflexologist.

Reflexology Techniques

Understanding a few of the basic reflexology techniques will help you get started.

- "Reflexing a point" means applying pressure to a specific area of the foot using a reflexology technique.

- "Walking" is one of the techniques used in reflexology to stimulate reflex points on the foot. It is done by using the outside edge of your thumb and walking across an area while maintaining contact with the skin and applying pressure each time you move your thumb forward. (You will benefit from either gentle or firm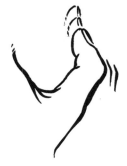

pressure.) You move your thumb forward by bending the thumb at the first joint (nearest your fingernail), keeping the rest of the thumb and its joints straight. The best way to understand what thumb-walking is like is to think of your thumb as an inchworm, inching its way up and down your foot. Sometimes walking is done with the fingers. Remember to take tiny steps.

Health note: Do not do reflexology on yourself, or have a treatment by a reflexologist, if you are recovering from surgery or are pregnant, or if you have diabetes, epilepsy, phlebitis or other blood-clotting conditions, a heart condition, an acute infection, or other serious medical conditions. If you have any of these conditions, are on medication, or have another health concern, consult with your doctor before receiving a reflexology treatment.[1]

Quick Fix Reflexology

Setting up the environment for reflexology can help you begin to focus your awareness on relaxing your mind and body, as well as prepare your feet for pampering. You can light candles, burn incense, or play soft music; whatever helps you feel calm and centered.

Reflexology is more comfortable and effective if the feet are warmed up and relaxed. Start your foot pampering with a foot soak to warm the feet and soften the skin, then give yourself a brief foot massage to loosen the muscles, tendons, and ligaments of the foot (see pages 53–59).

MINI REFLEXOLOGY TREATMENT

Generally, reflexologists reflex the left foot first before repeating the same steps and techniques on the right foot, but you can begin with either foot. Once you've completed the four steps on pages 70–76 on one foot, repeat the same sequence on your other foot.

ROTATE ANKLE

1. With the outside ankle of your left foot resting against your right thigh, support your left foot with your left hand.

2. Hold your heel, placing your right thumb on the spot between your ankle bone and the tip of your heel bone, and your index (or middle) finger on the same spot on the opposite (outside) side of your foot. Supporting and holding your toes with your left hand, gently rotate your foot in a clockwise direction several times. Repeat in counterclockwise direction.

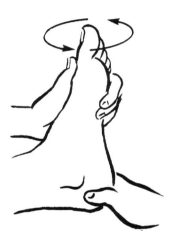

DOUBLE THUMB

1. With the outside ankle of your left foot resting against your right thigh, support your left foot with your left hand.

2. Holding both thumbs side by side, apply gentle pressure and slide thumbs up the arch of your foot, in between the pelvic and diaphragm lines. After you make a few passes, you can slowly increase the pressure if it feels comfortable.

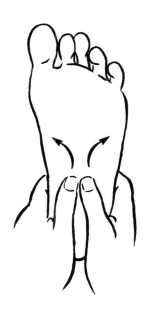

METATARSAL WAVE

1. With the outside ankle of your left foot resting against your right thigh, support your left foot with your left hand. You might want to sit next to another chair or couch for this step so that you can support your foot on the other chair and use both of your hands.

2. Placing both thumbs on the ball of your foot, gently squeeze the skin in the metatarsal area between your thumbs as you move back and forth across the metatarsal heads.

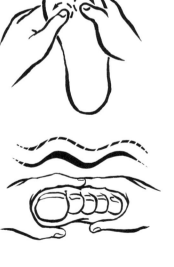

3. Keeping thumbs together, press thumbs on each side of a meta-tarsal joint and make alternating circles with your thumbs to move the joints. You can also hold each side of the foot and gently twist and undulate the ball of the foot (as if

you're creating a wave that moves from one side of the foot to the other) to loosen up the area.

SOLAR PLEXUS BREATHING

1. With the outside ankle of your left foot resting against your right thigh, support your left foot with your left hand.

2. Place the thumb of your left hand in the center of the spot where your arch turns into the ball of your foot (diaphragm line). As you press the point, take a deep breath. Hold the breath for a few seconds, then release it. As you release your breath, relax the pressure of your thumb against your foot. Repeat 3 times.

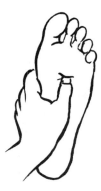

For those days when you feel especially tired or run-down, you can add two extra moves, clearing the zones and walking the spine.

CLEAR THE ZONES

The foot has five zones, each one running the length of the foot from each toe to the heel. Clearing the zones simply means using a reflexology technique called "walking" to reflex points along each zone.

1. With the outside ankle of your left foot resting against your right thigh, support your left foot with your left hand.

2. Begin with zone five (under the little toe). Using your right hand, walk your thumb in a straight line from the edge of your heel to the top of your little toe. Repeat with zone four (under fourth toe), zone three (under third toe), zone two (under second toe), and zone one (under big toe). When you've walked all five zones, repeat this sequence one more time.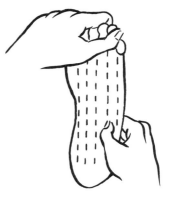

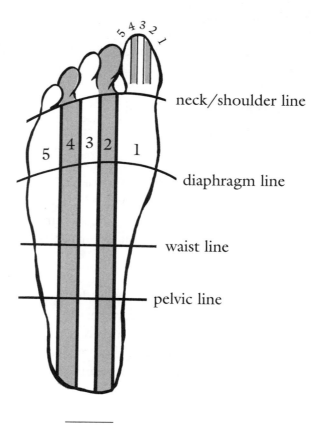

neck/shoulder line

diaphragm line

waist line

pelvic line

WALK THE SPINE

In this step, you'll be using the walking technique described on pages 67–68.

1. With the outside ankle of your left foot resting against your right thigh, support your left foot with your left hand.

2. With your right hand, walk your thumb along the inside edge of your foot, from heel to top of big toe. Then walk along the inside edge of your foot, from the top of the big toe to the heel.

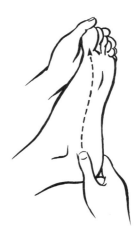

You can end your session by reflexing points on your feet (see reflexology map). Press each point for 5 to 30 seconds, depending on what feels comfortable for you. Different points on your feet may feel tender, but if any feel painful, stop pressing. Don't worry about moving up or down or across; just press all over the bottoms of your feet.

Example: After a long day, you might want to squeeze each of your toes (with thumb on toe pad and finger on toenail) between your thumb and forefinger. Then you can walk the different areas: balls of feet, arches, heels, and ankles.

SELF-MASSAGE TOOLS & TOYS

For quick pick-me-ups, keep some of these reflexology and massage tools and toys in your desk drawer at work or in a handy spot at home. These products can stimulate, revitalize, and massage the feet in just a few minutes, and they can be used several times throughout the day. You can find these products at massage supply stores, bath and herbal shops, and even at some drugstores. Here are a few of my favorites:

WOODEN FOOT ROLLER

Instructions: Sitting in a comfortable, supportive chair, slip off your shoes and roll the foot roller back and forth underneath your right foot for several minutes. Repeat with left foot. You can also use a nubby foot roller.

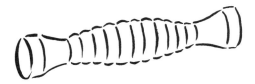

ROLLING WOODEN BALLS

Instructions: Sitting in a comfortable and supportive chair, slip off your shoes and run your right foot back and forth against the balls for several minutes. Repeat with left foot.

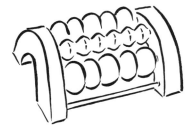

Nubby Ball

Nubby balls combine reflexology, acupuncture, and massage to stimulate reflex points on your feet.

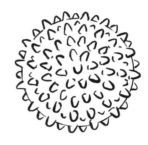

Instructions: Sitting in a comfortable and supportive chair, slip off your shoes and socks. Place a nubby ball under your left foot and roll the ball up and down, from your heel to your toes. Then roll the ball against the arch of your foot in a circular motion. Roll the ball against your heel, ball of foot, and toes. Roll it across all parts of your foot. Repeat with right foot. If you're coordinated, you can use a ball under each foot at the same time. Try to maintain an even pressure.

Thumb Massagers

Thumb massagers are plastic thumb shoes with nubs on the bottom; they also combine reflexology, acupuncture, and massage to stimulate reflex points on your feet.

Instructions: Sitting in a comfortable and supportive chair, slip off your shoes and socks. Wearing thumb massagers, walk your thumbs along the bottom of your left foot, from heel to base of toes. Repeat several times, covering entire bottom of foot. Walk around your ankles, then along the arch of your foot. Then, holding foot with one hand, walk thumb up each toe, squeezing the tips of your toes between your thumb and forefinger. Repeat on right foot.

Reflexology Socks

Reflexology socks have reflexology maps printed on them so you can find all the reflex points without looking at a book.

5 Foot Fitness

Keep the faculty of effort alive in you by a little gratuitous exercise every day.

—WILLIAM JAMES

In addition to maintaining a well-rounded fitness plan that includes cardiovascular training for 20–30 minutes every day, strength training for 20 minutes at least twice a week, and regular flexibility exercises like stretching or yoga, you need to exercise your feet, too. Walking is the best exercise for your feet and calves, and adding a few stretching and strengthening exercises to your daily routine will help keep the muscles of your feet, toes, ankles, and lower legs flexible and strong.

STRONG BODY, STRONG FEET

The exercises in this section are divided into three categories:

1. *Foot stretches* are meant to stretch the muscles, ligaments, and tendons of the feet. For best results, these stretches should be done daily.

2. *Strengthening exercises* are meant to strengthen the muscles of the feet and ankles. (Including a few *advanced ankle exercises,* for athletes or other people who have mastered the basic exercises and want a more challenging workout.) Practice these exercises three to five times a week.

3. *Toe exercises* are meant to exercise the toes, lubricate the toe joints, stretch the arches of the feet, and increase toe dexterity. For best results, these exercises should be done daily.

Before You Begin

Here are a few guidelines to keep in mind when stretching and exercising your feet and lower legs.

Tips:
- Ease into the exercises and stretches slowly and gently. You may want to go for a short walk to warm up your muscles, or soak your feet in warm water, before you begin.

- Unless noted, exercises should be done barefoot for better traction with the floor.

- During balancing exercises you may want to stand close to a wall, or use the back of a chair, in case you need some extra support.

- In general, stretches should be held for 30 seconds. If holding for 30 seconds is too difficult, hold for 20 or 10 seconds, and gradually work up to 30 seconds.

- If you are already working with a doctor, podiatrist, trainer, or physical therapist, consult with her/him before trying these exercises to make sure that they are appropriate for you.

Rating: Some of the exercises are rated I (safe for most people) or II (more challenging), but you are the best judge of what feels comfortable to you.

HealthNotes:

- Do not do any exercises that are painful for you.

- If you have diminished balance, do not do any of the balancing postures without supervision.

- If you have foot problems like bunions, arthritis, or diabetes, ask your doctor if these exercises are appropriate for you, and ask for modifications of the exercises that seem too difficult for you.

- As with any physical exercise, you should consult your doctor before beginning a new exercise routine.

FOOT STRETCHES

Ankle Exercise

Benefits:

This is a good exercise to begin with to gently loosen up the muscles that support the ankle. The motion lubricates the joint and prepares the foot and lower leg for movement.

Instructions:

1. Sit in a supportive chair with your feet placed on the floor, directly below your knees (your upper and lower leg should form a 90-degree angle).

2. Lifting your right foot off the floor, extend your right leg, keeping your knee slightly bent.

3. Rotate your right foot in a clockwise direction 20 times, then rotate your foot in a counterclockwise direction 20 times. Repeat with left foot.

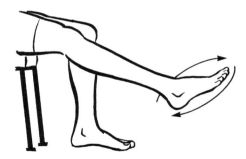

Rating: I

Standing Foot Stretch

Benefits:

Stretches the toes and the muscles on the tops and bottoms of feet.

Instructions:

1. Stand still, with head held high, abs slightly engaged, knees slightly bent, arms hanging loosely at your sides, eyes looking straight ahead.

2. Take your right foot and press the tops of your toes gently into the floor. You will feel a stretch across the top of your foot and the front of your ankle. Hold for 30 seconds. Repeat with other foot.

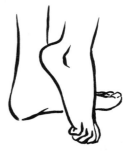

3. Take your right foot and flex your toes against the floor while lifting your heel off of the floor. You will feel a stretch across the bottom of your foot and through your arch. Hold for 30 seconds. Repeat with other foot. Repeat exercise 3–5 times.

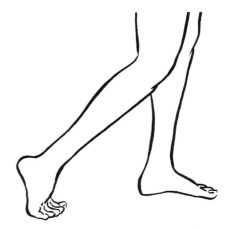

Tips:
- You may have to bend the knee of your standing leg and move your active leg around until you can find a foot placement that gives you the best stretch.

- Don't hold your breath; keep breathing.

- Practice next to a wall, or use the back of a chair for support, if you feel unsteady.

Rating: I

Calf Stretch

Benefits:

Stretching the calf muscles is an important element of foot care. If your calves are tight, your Achilles tendon can become tight too, which in turn can make the muscles in the arch of the foot tight, resulting in heel pain. Stretching the calf muscles also stretches the Achilles tendon. These stretches are good for people suffering from plantar fasciitis and/or heel pain.

Instructions:

1. Standing 5 or 6 inches away from a wall, place your hands on the wall at chest level. Move your left leg back 1 or 2 feet. Bend your right leg slightly, and place toes of right foot a few inches away from the wall. Keep your back leg straight. Don't forget to maintain good posture during this stretch. Your head, neck, back, hips, left knee, and left ankle should form a straight line.

2. Lean into the wall, keeping both heels on the floor. You will feel the stretch in the back of your extended leg. Hold for 30–60 seconds. Repeat with other foot. Repeat sequence 3–5 times.

3. Do the stretch again, but this time with your extended back leg slightly bent. You will feel this stretch lower down on the back of your leg. Hold for 30–60 seconds. Repeat with other leg. Repeat sequence 3–5 times.

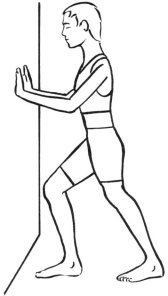

Tips:

- Remember to keep heels on the floor.

- Upper body should not lean into the wall, but the pelvis should move forward toward the wall.

- Do this stretch slowly, and don't push yourself too hard. If you feel pain, you're stretching too far, and you should stop.

Rating: I

Incline Stretch

Benefits:

Stretching your calf muscle and Achilles tendon is good for overall foot health and stability. This is a good stretch for people suffering from plantar fasciitis and/or heel pain.

Instructions:

1. Use a foam-wedge Slant Board or a Multi-Slant Board with adjustable incline levels for this stretch, or make your own incline by placing a thin piece of wood (1 inch thick or less, 1 foot long, wide enough to accommodate your foot) against a block of wood.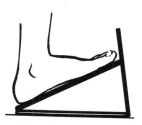

2. Place your right foot on the incline, putting your weight into your heel. You will feel the stretch in your Achilles tendon, which is the area behind your ankle, rising from your heel up to your calf. Hold for 30–60 seconds. Repeat for other foot. Repeat stretch 3–5 times.

Tip:
• If you are very flexible and you don't feel much of a stretch, you may need to increase the incline of the stretch. Start with the lower height first, though, to avoid over-stretching.

Rating: I

Health Notes:

• Stretch with awareness. Don't push yourself into pain.

• People with diminished balance should be very careful practicing this stretch.

Plantar Flexion/Dorsiflexion

In this exercise you will practice plantar flexion (extending toes away from body) and ankle dorsiflexion (extending heel and pointing toes toward face). This is a good alternative for people who find toe raises too difficult.

Benefits:

Stretches and limbers the ankle muscles and the Achilles tendon.

Instructions:

1. Lie on your back with arms at sides and ankles together. Take a few deep, slow breaths to relax your body.

2. Point toes away from body, reaching with toes as if you might touch the opposite wall. Hold for 30 seconds. Relax feet and let go of the stretch.

3. Point toes toward your nose, reaching with toes for the wall behind you. Hold for 30 seconds. Relax feet and let go of the stretch. Repeat sequence.

Rating: I

STRENGTHENING EXERCISES

These strengthening exercises are often used in ankle rehabilitation; they're great for strengthening the muscles that help stabilize the foot and the ankle joint.

For these exercises, you will need an exercise band, a thin, wide strap of rubber used in physical therapy exercises. Exercise bands, which can be found at massage supply stores, usually come in a variety of colors, with each color corresponding to a

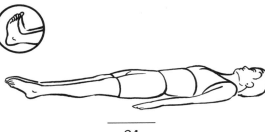

different resistance level. Your band should be about 3 to 5 feet long. You want the band to be long enough to hold both ends in your hand when you are in a seated position and the band is looped around your foot. For best results, complete all four exercises in succession.

Calf and Ankle Strengtheners

Benefits:

This is a very gentle way to begin strengthening the calf muscles, and an ideal exercise for people new to exercise, older people, or people recovering from an injury. These four exercises help strengthen the ankles and improve range of motion.

Calf and Ankle Strength I

Instructions:

1. Sit in a supportive chair with your feet placed on the floor, directly below your knees (your upper and lower leg

should form a 90-degree angle). You can sit on the floor if it's more comfortable for you.

2. Extend your right foot a few inches off the ground, keeping your knee slightly bent. Place the middle of the band

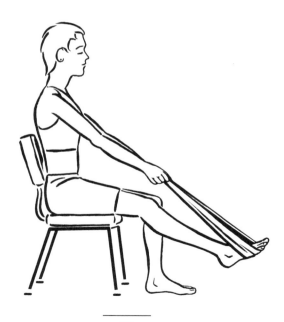

around the ball of your foot and hold on to the ends of the band with your hands. (You can also bring the ends together and hold them in one hand.)

3. Against the resistance of the band, slowly press against the band as if you are pressing on the gas pedal of a car. Hold your foot in that extended position for several seconds. Release slowly, maintaining tension in the band. Repeat 10–15 times. Rest. Repeat on left foot. Then repeat the sequence 2 more times.

Tip:

- For all of the band exercises, you want to maintain tension on the band when pushing against the band and when releasing it so that the foot can move through its maximum comfort range in both directions.

Rating: I

Calf and Ankle Strength 2

Instructions:

1. Place your chair in front of a heavy piece of furniture, like a table or bed. Sit in a supportive chair with your feet placed on the floor, directly below your knees (your upper and lower leg should form a 90-degree angle). For a greater range of motion in this exercise, sit on the floor instead of in a chair.

2. Loop the band around the leg of a heavy table or bed, then tie the ends in a knot. Place your right foot in the loop so that the band runs across the top of your foot (your right leg will no longer be at a 90-degree angle).

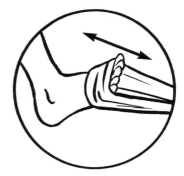

3. Against the resistance of the band, slowly pull the top of your foot toward your body, leaving your heel on the floor. Hold your foot in that upright position for several seconds. Release slowly. Repeat 10–15 times. Rest. Repeat on left foot. Then repeat the sequence 2 more times.

Tips:

- If you're ready for a more challenging calf-strengthening exercise, see Toe Raises on pages 103–104.

- For all of the band exercises, make sure that the furniture you use is heavy enough to stay firmly in place when you do each exercise.

Rating: I

Ankle Strength 1

Instructions:

1. Sit in a supportive chair with your feet placed on the floor, directly below your knees (your upper and lower leg should form a 90-degree angle). You can sit on the floor if it's more comfortable for you.

2. Loop your band around the leg of a heavy table or bed, then tie the ends in a knot. The band should then be lying on the floor to the right of the table leg. Place your right foot into the loop so that the right side of your foot is cradled in the band. You may have to adjust your chair so that the band is parallel with your chair.

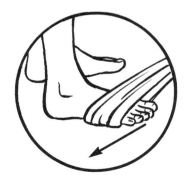

3. Against the resistance of the band, press the side of your foot into the band, pulling it away from the table leg. Your heel should remain on the floor, and your forefoot should be as close to the floor as possible. Hold the extended position for several seconds. Release slowly. Repeat 10–15 times. Rest. Repeat on left foot. Then repeat the sequence 2 more times.

Rating: I

Ankle Strength 2

Instructions:

1. Sit in a supportive chair with your feet placed on the floor, directly below your knees (your upper and lower leg should form a 90-degree angle). You can sit on the floor if it's more comfortable for you.

2. Loop the band around the leg of a heavy table or bed, then tie the ends in a knot. The band should then be lying on the floor to the left of the table leg.

3. Place your right foot into the loop so that the left side of your foot is cradled in the band. You may have to adjust your chair so that the band is parallel with your chair.

4. Against the resistance of the band, press the side of your foot into the band, pulling it away from the table leg. Your heel should remain on the floor, and your forefoot should be as close to the floor as possible. Hold that position for several seconds. Release slowly. Repeat 10–15 times. Rest. Repeat on left foot. Then repeat the sequence 2 more times.

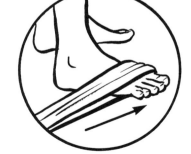

Rating: I

OTHER STRENGTHENING EXERCISES

Toe Raises

Benefits:

Strengthens calf muscles.

Instructions:

1. Stand on the first step of a staircase, holding the handrail for balance.

2. Edge your feet slowly off the step until you are balancing on the balls of your feet and your toes.

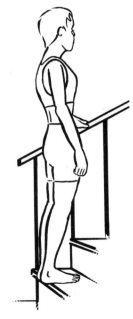

3. Slowly raise yourself on your toes. Pause, then lower your heels toward the floor for maximal stretch. Pause, then raise up on your toes again so that you complete a full range of motion. Repeat sequence 10–15 times.

Tips:

- If you feel strong enough, you can do this exercise using one foot while holding the other foot slightly away from your body to the side or behind you so that it's not touching the step. Then repeat with opposite foot.

- For best results, do this exercise at least three times a week.

Rating: I or II

Health Note:

This exercise is not recommended for anyone with diminished balance, big toe problems, or plantar fasciitis.

Rocker Board Ankle Mobility Exercise

Benefits:

Exercising with a rocker, or "wobble" board, can increase ankle strength and range of motion, and improve flexibility and balance.

Instructions:

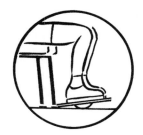

1. Sit in a supportive, comfortable chair. Place your feet on the board, parallel and near the edges of the board.

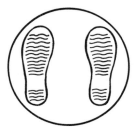

2. Make a circle with the board against the floor, pressing the edge of the board into the floor as you rotate it. Continue exercise for 1–3 minutes. Repeat, rotating board in opposite direction.

3. Repeat exercise with feet parallel on board, but moved closer to the center of the board. Continue for 1–3 minutes. Repeat, rotating board in opposite direction.

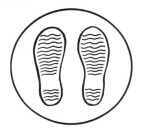

Tips:

• Board should be used on a carpeted floor.

• Wear rubber-soled shoes for the best traction.

• Edges of board should remain in contact with the floor during exercise.

• For best results, do this exercise at least 3 times a week.

Rating: I

Rocker Board Strengthening Exercise

This exercise is similar to the previous one but is done standing.

1. Stand in a doorway. Holding the edges of the doorway for support, stand on the board with feet parallel and near the edges of the board.

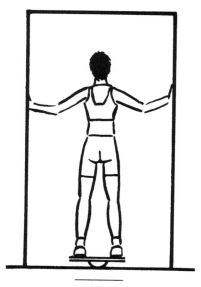

2. Make a circle with the board against the floor, pressing the edge of the board into the floor as you rotate it. Continue exercises for 1–3 minutes. Repeat, rotating board in opposite direction.

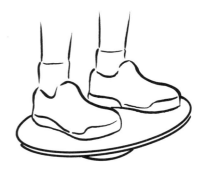

3. Repeat exercise with feet parallel on board, but moved closer to the center of the board. Continue for 1–3 minutes. Repeat, rotating board in opposite direction.

4. Repeat exercise with one foot placed on the center of the board. Continue for 1–3 minutes. Repeat, rotating board in opposite direction. Repeat with other foot.

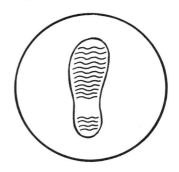

Tips:

- Only do this exercise in a doorway where you can hold on to the edges for support.

- Board should be used on a carpeted floor.

- Wear rubber-soled shoes for the best traction.

- Edges of board should remain in contact with the floor during exercise.

- For best results, do this exercise at least 3 times a week.

Rating: II

Health Note:

Not recommended for people with diminished balance.

THE LITTLE FOOT CARE BOOK

FIVE TOE TRICKS

Strengthening the toes can help prevent foot problems. These five exercises, recommended by the American Orthopaedic Foot and Ankle Society (AOFAS), can be done daily. As with all stretching and strengthening exercises in this book, try to maintain your natural alignment and posture during exercises.

If you have bunions or other foot problems that make these exercises difficult, or if any of the exercises cause pain, ask your doctor or physical therapist to recommend modifications of these exercises, or other exercises, for you.

Toe Pulls and Big Toe Press

Benefits:

Good for preventing bunions, hammertoes, and toe cramps.

Instructions:

1. Place a thick rubber band around all of your toes, and then spread toes apart, stretching the rubber band. Hold for 5 seconds. Repeat 10 times. If you can't find a rubber band that fits, just spread toes apart, hold, repeat. Also, stretch the rubber band between your big toes, keeping heels in place on the floor.

2. Next, with feet parallel and about an inch apart, try to touch the upper, outside edges of your big toes together without moving your feet or other toes. Hold for 5 seconds. Release. Repeat 10 times.

*If you have bunions, these exercises might be very difficult for you.

Ball Roll

Benefits:

Massages arch of foot. Good for plantar fasciitis, arch strain, heel pain, and foot cramps.

Instructions:

Massage the bottom of your foot by rolling a golf ball or a tennis ball (if the ball's a bit flat, all the better) under the arch and ball of your foot for two minutes. Repeat with opposite foot.

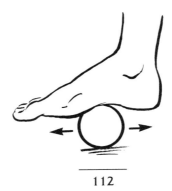

Towel Scrunches

Benefits:

Good for hammertoes, toe cramps, pain in ball of foot.

Instructions:

1. Sit in a supportive chair with your feet flat on the floor, knees aligned over your ankles (i.e., upper and lower legs forming a 90-degree angle). Place a towel at the edge of the toes of your right foot.

2. Slowly grasp the towel, pulling it toward you with the toes of your right foot until you reach the other end of the towel. (Your upper and lower legs may not remain in a 90-degree angle). Repeat 5 times. Repeat with left foot. To make this exercise a bit more difficult, place a weight or a can of soup on the end of the towel.

ABCs

Benefits:

Strengthens and exercises foot and toes.

Instructions:

Sitting in a comfortable, supportive chair, extend your right leg, keeping your knee bent, and trace the letters of the alphabet against the floor with your big toe. Repeat with opposite foot.

Walk in Sand

Benefits:

Massages, exfoliates, and strengthens toes. Strengthens leg muscles.

Instructions:

Walking barefoot in dry sand massages your feet, strengthens your toes, and exfoliates the dry skin on the bottoms of your feet.

Health Note:

Running barefoot in the sand is not recommended because of the increased risk of overstretching calf muscles and injuring muscles and tendons.

6 If the Shoe Fits

You cannot put the same shoe on every foot.
                              —PUBLILIUS SYRUS

According to the American Podiatric Medical Association, 80 percent of us will experience foot problems in our lifetimes, and two-thirds of those problems will be caused by poorly fitting shoes. Women are especially at risk of developing foot problems because they are more likely than men to wear narrow, tapered shoes, not to mention high heels. Bunions, bunionettes, neuromas, and hammertoes are the most common problems caused by poorly fitting shoes, and women have 90 percent of the 795,000 annual surgeries to address those problems.[1]

In a survey of 356 women, the AOFAS found that 90 percent were wearing shoes too small for their feet, and 80 percent of those women had foot problems. Most of the women in the study had not had their feet measured in more than five years. Some of the most common conditions caused by improperly fitting dress shoes are calluses and corns, bunions and hammertoes, and blisters.

The bottom line is, if you wear shoes that are too small (or too big) for your feet, you're probably going to develop foot problems. You might start off with blisters or sore feet, but you can end up damaging muscles, joints, and bones.

TEN SHOE-FITTING TIPS

1. Shop at stores that have experienced shoe fitters who can help you find shoe styles appropriate for your specific foot characteristics and activity needs. Sometimes smaller independent shoe stores (and shoe stores in department stores) have better customer service and more experienced salespeople than large chain stores.

2. Shop for shoes at the end of the day when your feet are largest, and wear the type of socks you're most likely to wear with your new shoes.

3. Ask the salesperson to measure both feet (length and width; measurement should be taken while you are standing), as well as take an arch measurement. Even though shoe sizes vary from brand to brand and may not correspond exactly to your measurements, having your feet measured is still important because the measurements give the salesperson a better idea of your foot shape.

   Select a shoe that fits your arch, as well as the length and width of your foot. The ball of your foot should fit in the widest part of the shoe, and you should have a ⅜ to ½ inch space between your longest toe and the end of your shoe (when standing). You should have enough room to wiggle your toes. Shoe width should match your foot to within ¼ inch. Most people have one foot that's slightly larger than the other; buy shoes to fit the largest foot.

4. Don't worry about size, and don't shop by brand. Just because you've always worn a size 7 doesn't mean you always will. Sizes are rarely consistent among brands, and your feet get larger with age (and during pregnancy). Within each brand, companies may have some shoes that are good for your feet and some that don't fit your feet. Buy what feels comfortable.

5. Select shoes that are wide enough to accommodate your feet. This is particularly important for women, because so many styles are harmful to women's feet. If the shoes you try on are too narrow, ask if they come in a wider width. If they don't, try on another style. Don't let the salesperson convince you that going up a size will take care of the width.

   Take the shoe test to avoid being tempted by tiny shoes:

Stand on a piece of paper and trace the outline of your foot. When you get to the shoe store, place the tracing under whichever shoes you like. If the shoes are smaller than the tracing, don't even try them on; they are too narrow for your feet.

In general, look for shoes that are available in different widths, but don't forget to look for a shoe that also conforms to your foot shape. Buying a wide shoe that's built on a last that doesn't fit your foot won't solve the problem. For example, you might have a wide forefoot but a narrow heel, or you might have high arches. You want to find a shoe that fits all of your foot characteristics.

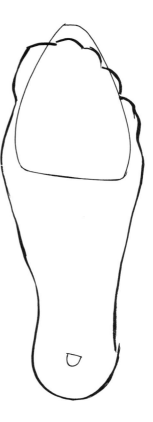

6. Shoes don't stretch. If they feel too tight in the store, get a bigger size. You should not have to "break in" shoes to have them fit properly. They should feel comfortable as soon as you put them on. If the salesperson offers to stretch a shoe to make it fit, don't buy it. You should walk out of the store with shoes that fit when you put them on.

7. Your heel should fit comfortably in the heel counter. If your heel slips or feels pinched when you walk, try a different size or another style.

8. Check for any seams or pieces of material inside the shoes that could irritate your feet.

9. Walk around the store for several minutes to get a feel for how the shoes fit.

10. Buy quality shoes that fit well. Well-made shoes will last longer, especially if you don't wear the same pair of shoes every day, and can often be repaired and resoled. (Be aware that expensive shoes aren't always high quality.) Cheap shoes don't last very long, and they could hurt

your feet. Also, avoid inexpensive knockoffs of popular brands. They might look similar to the more expensive shoes, but they almost always lack the technology, engineering, and quality materials that make the more expensive shoes good for your feet.

You may spend $150–$350 for a good pair of shoes or boots, but it's money well spent, and in the long run, quality shoes are a bargain if they help you avoid bunion surgery, or other foot-related medical bills, in the future.

WHAT TO LOOK FOR IN A SHOE

You don't have to be a shoe scientist to find a good pair of shoes, but it is worth reviewing these guidelines to give yourself an idea of which features to look for the next time you need new shoes.

- *Breathability:* Look for shoes with uppers (the top part of the shoe that surrounds your foot) made out of breathable material like leather, suede, or canvas. Avoid shoes made out of synthetic materials.

- *Cushioning:* Consider that a 150-pound person exerts a pressure of 63.5 tons on their feet just from walking one mile.[2] Shoes that have good cushioning (in the soles, mid-soles, and heel cup) can help absorb some of that impact. Beware of shoes with too much cushioning; they might not provide adequate support. If the shoes feel wobbly when you walk, they don't have enough support.

- *Soles:* The soles of your shoes should be appropriate for the surfaces on which you will be walking (or running, hiking, playing sports, and so on). Avoid thin-soled, flat, or slip-on shoes, which generally don't have adequate cushioning or support. Heel height should be no greater than 1 inch.

- *Stability:* Your shoes should support your feet. Look for well-constructed shoes made by reputable shoe companies. Before you try on a shoe, inspect it for stability: Squeeze the heel counter of the shoe. The firmer it is, the better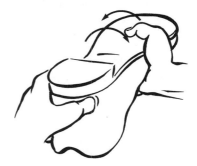

support it will provide. Turn the shoe upside down in your hands. Hold the heel in one hand and the sole (at the ball of the foot area of the shoe) in the other. Twist the shoe from side to side. The harder it is to twist, the more stability and support the shoe will provide from the heel to the ball of the foot. It's okay if the toe of the shoe is soft enough to flex back and forth. You want a little bit of flexibility in the forefoot.

- *Shape:* Buy shoes that most closely conform to the shape of your foot. Companies make their shoes based on lasts, which are basically models of different sizes and shapes of feet. The last on which a shoe is built determines its fit characteristics. Some lasts have a narrow heel and a wide forefoot. Some lasts have rounded toes, or pointed toes. Other lasts have more depth throughout the arch and toe box.

  Shoes are made on thousands of different lasts. Even within one company, each style can be made on a different last. That's why sometimes you find a shoe that fits, but another style in the same brand doesn't fit well. What makes shoe buying difficult is that you don't know what type of last the shoe was made on, which makes it important for you and the shoe fitter who helps you to find shoes that match the shape of your foot.

Shoes that have a rounded toe box generally provide the best fit for most feet. Avoid narrow, pointed, high-heeled shoes that push the feet into unnatural positions.

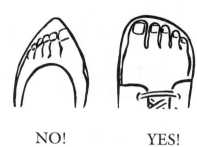

NO!   YES!

WHY HIGH HEELS ARE BAD FOR YOU

• Wearing high heels can shorten the Achilles tendon over time, causing heel pain and decreased range of motion. Seventy-five percent of the 2 million Americans that suffer from heel pain are women.[3]

• High heels force the weight of the body forward, placing 90 percent of your body weight over the balls of the feet. This added pressure to the forefeet increases your risk of forefoot injury, and it throws off body alignment.[4]

- High-heeled shoes have narrow, pointed toe boxes that cramp the toes and forefeet, contributing to foot problems like corns, hammertoes, and bunions.

- Eight out of ten women develop foot problems from wearing high heels on a regular basis.[5]

A CLOSET FULL OF SHOES

It's impossible to recommend shoes by brand, since everyone's feet are unique. Even the many shoe salespeople, podiatrists, orthopedic surgeons, physical therapists, and pedorthists I talked to during my research were reluctant to name brands. However, there were a few names (for a variety of budgets) that came up repeatedly, many of which I have worn, so I have listed those shoes under each of the following categories. Please keep in mind that the best shoe for you is the shoe that fits. If your favorite shoes are not listed here, that does not mean that they aren't right for you. The brands listed here are merely suggestions to give you an idea of the many options you have when shopping for shoes. Many of the brands listed make women's and men's shoes.

Dress/Work Shoes

It's always difficult to find the perfect black shoes to match your perfect black dress (never mind comfort), but with all the shoe companies out there, you should be able to combine fashion and comfort. Mephisto, Theresia, Think!, Paul Green, and Donald J. Pliner all make high-quality, fashionable dress shoes designed with comfort in mind. If you're looking for something elegant, yet comfortable, to match an evening dress, Taryn Rose makes a variety of dressy styles. Moderate to lower-priced dress shoes include Beautifeel, Munro, Selby, and Naked Feet (which feature contoured footbeds and funky designs). For dress casual, Birkenstock, Finn Comfort, Easy Spirit, and Naturalizer make styles with deeper and rounded toe boxes. For men: Finn Comfort, Dino Monti, Birkenstock, Mephisto, Think!, Stonefly, and Donald J. Pliner.

Athletic Shoes and Walking Shoes

With all the choices out there, it can be difficult to decide on an athletic shoe, especially when it seems as if new styles appear in the stores every few months. Although today's athletic shoes are much better designed and constructed than the sneakers you wore as a child, sophisticated technology and flashy colors don't always translate into good fit. New Balance is the only athletic shoe company that makes a full line of shoes from AA to EE widths for women and B to EEEE for men. Other athletic shoe companies, like Asics and Adidas, make some of their top-selling styles in two different widths.

Tips:
- Ask your doctor, physical therapist, and other athletes to recommend good shoe stores.

- For comfort and injury prevention, buy sport-specific athletic shoes. If you don't play any sports but just want a general athletic shoe for a variety of activities, a cross-training shoe might be appropriate for you.

- Athletic shoes are predominantly made out of synthetic materials. After your activity, return to wearing leather shoes, which provide better breathability.

Keep in mind that everybody's feet are different, and you might need more or less of one feature than the next person. For example, a runner who pronates might need a different type of running shoe than does another runner who has trouble with shin splints. To reduce the risk of injury, make sure you buy the shoes that fit your foot type and activity.

Here are some general features that the AOFAS recommends in different athletic shoes:

- Walking shoes should provide cushioning/shock absorption in the heel and forefoot, a rocker-bottom sole (i.e., a slightly rounded sole that helps the shoe shift weight between the heels to the toes with each step).

- Aerobics shoes should provide cushioning/shock absorption in the forefoot.

- Running shoes should provide cushioning/shock absorption in the heel and forefoot, stability, heel control. Runners should replace their shoes every 350–500 miles.[6]

- Tennis shoes should provide support during side-to-side movements, stability, flexibility. On soft courts: a sole with better traction. On hard courts: a sole with better tread.

- Basketball shoes should provide a thick, stiff sole, cushioning, high top for ankle support.

- Cross-training shoes should provide flexibility in forefoot, stability.

On its website, the AOFAS also recommends different lacing techniques that can help you in fitting athletic shoes.

Although styles and style names may change each year, checking out shoe reviews in magazines like *Health, Walking, Backpacker, Runner's World,* and other sport-specific magazines might help you identify shoes that you might want to try on when shopping.

Comfort Shoes

"Comfort shoes" have become more popular as people realize that the shoes they wear impact their foot health and comfort. Look for stores that specialize in walking and comfort shoes for everyday wear and for work. Some of the brands you might see there (for men and women) include Mephisto, Finn Comfort, Clark's, Stonefly, Ecco, Wolky's, Naot, Reiker, Josef Seibel, Dansko, and Birkenstock.

HARD-TO-FIT FEET

If you have a hard time finding shoes that fit, you're not alone. Many people, whether they have foot problems or not, have hard-to-fit feet. Maybe your feet are long and narrow, or short and wide. Maybe high or low arches make some shoes uncomfortable for you. Or maybe you have a combination of foot characteristics that makes finding shoes difficult. An experienced shoe fitter should be able to help you find a style that's comfortable. If you still need help, your doctor should be able to refer you to someone who can recommend some brands and styles of shoes that might work for you. You can also try some of the brands listed in the comfort and orthotic sections.

Injuries and Disease

If you have an injury or disease that makes it hard to find shoes that fit, your doctor might refer you to an orthotist (usually a physical therapist trained in orthotic fabrication or a podiatrist) or a pedorthist (a foot-care specialist trained and certified in shoe modification, anatomy of the foot, physiology and biomechanics, and orthotic fabrication).

The goal of pedorthists is to unite the foot, shoe, and orthotic to help alleviate foot problems caused by injury or disease. Sometimes simple modifications to shoes and/or wearing custom-made orthotics can make a big difference. Pedorthists can often help people with chronic pain, foot deformities caused by bunions or arthritis, diabetes, or other special needs get back on their feet again. To find out more about pedorthics, or to find a pedorthist in your area, check out the Pedorthic Footwear Association's website at www.pedorthics.org.

Wide and Narrow Feet

With so many styles of shoes available, you should be able to find shoes that are the right width for you. Again, your shoe fitter should be able to recommend brands that come in different widths. Rockport makes dress, casual, and outdoor shoes for women and men in a range of sizes and widths. Women with wide feet can also wear men's or boy's shoes.

Orthotic Wearer

If you wear orthotics, put them in any shoes you try on at the store.

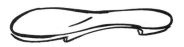

Buy the size that fits when you're wearing your orthotics. You may have to buy your shoes a half-size larger, or wider, to accommodate your orthotics. Look for extra-depth shoes that have room for orthotics.

The insoles in most athletic and casual shoes can be removed so that your shoe can accommodate a full-length orthotic. Most people who need orthotics have one pair for sports shoes and another pair for everyday shoes. In some cases, you may need more than two pairs.

Orthopedic shoe brands like Drew and PW Minor make shoes in widths, as well as shoes with a wide forefoot and narrow heel. They also come in deeper toe-box styles to accommodate orthotics and feet with bunions and hammertoes. Comfort shoes like Finn Comfort and Birkenstock come with removable, modifiable, contoured cork footbeds that can sometimes eliminate the need for custom-made orthotics.

SOCKS

Wearing the right socks can be as important as wearing the right shoes. A good pair of socks can protect your feet in many ways: they reduce the friction and rubbing between your feet and the insides of your shoes, they absorb moisture from the feet, and they keep your feet warm in cold weather.

As with shoes, you want to buy socks that fit well and that are appropriate for the shoes you'll be wearing and for the activities in which they'll be worn. Socks that are too small can constrict your feet, and socks that are too big can bunch up in your shoe, causing blisters. Look for socks with a heel pocket; they are more comfortable and fit better than "tube" socks that have no defined heel and can slip around on the feet. High-quality socks will have defined heel and toe pockets for the best fit, as well as extra reinforcement in these areas to make the socks last longer. Avoid socks that are too tight around the feet, ankles, or lower legs, or have any seams in the toe area that irritate your toes.

For everyday wear, socks made out of natural fibers like cotton and wool are good for the skin, allow the foot to breathe, and absorb moisture. You should change your socks at least once a day; walking around in soggy socks can increase your chances of getting athlete's foot and/or blisters. Avoid nylons, which don't let the feet breathe. If you have a problem with excessively sweaty feet, you might want to wear socks made out of technical fibers that have a better wicking capability than cotton.

Wearing the appropriate socks during your recreational activities can also help you keep your feet comfortable and prevent skin problems. In general, you'll want to look for socks made out of synthetic fibers like acrylic, nylon, spandex, polyester, and polypropylene, or a blend of synthetic fibers and cotton or wool, for sports and other vigorous activities because they'll keep your feet drier. Both Wigwam and Thorlos make a wide range of high-quality dress and athletic socks.

7 When Feet Go Bad

When our feet hurt, we hurt all over.
                        —SOCRATES

YOUR ACHING FEET

If you have foot problems, you're not alone. Seventy-five million Americans currently have foot problems,[1] and each year 54 million Americans, or one out of five people, will have a foot problem.[2] Sixty-two percent of men and women who participated in a Dr. Scholl's foot health survey said that their feet hurt regularly, and that they expected them to hurt.

What most people don't understand is that foot pain is not normal.

Most foot ailments are caused by neglect, poorly fitting shoes, and injuries. Just as you brush your teeth every day to prevent cavities, practicing preventive foot care measures can reduce the number and severity of many common foot problems. If you already have a foot problem, like dry skin, calluses, or bunions, learning more about it can help you get the medical attention you need. It's always better to address minor foot problems before they become major problems; you'll have more conservative treatment options available to you.

This section of the book is meant to help you become more familiar with some of the most common foot problems so that you can try to prevent them. It should not be a substitute for seeking a diagnosis and treatment from your physician.

Health note: If you are pregnant or have an existing medical condition, especially in the cases of diabetes, epilepsy, or heart or circulatory problems, consult your doctor before considering any of the self-care suggestions in this book.

Who Can Help You

If you have any concerns about your feet, see your doctor. Your regular doctor can treat your foot problems, and in some cases may refer you to foot specialists. Here are some of the people who can help you take care of your feet:

- **Orthopedic surgeons** are medical doctors (M.D.'s) who treat injuries, deformities, and diseases of the musculoskeletal system. Their training includes four years of medical school, a year-long surgery internship, and at least four years of a hospital surgery residency. Orthopedists who specialize in foot and ankle surgery also spend an extra year completing special surgical training.

- **Podiatrists** are doctors of podiatric medicine (D.P.M.'s) who treat all foot problems. Their training includes four years of podiatric medical college. The majority of podiatrists also complete at least one to three years of hospital residency, which includes surgical training. Podiatrists are also trained in biomechanical evaluation and orthotic fabrication.

- **Physical therapists** are licensed health care providers (B.S.P.T. or M.S.P.T.) who help restore function to the body after injury or illness. Their training includes four years of physical therapy school, or a master's program after completing a four-year college degree.

- **Dermatologists** are medical doctors (M.D.'s) who specialize in disorders of the skin. Their training includes four years of medical school, a one-year medical or surgical internship, and a three-year residency in dermatology (longer for those who study a specialty). Dermatologists treat a variety of foot problems, including athlete's foot, plantar warts, toenail fungus, dry skin, and rashes.

- **Orthotists and pedorthists** are trained and certified in the fabrication and fitting of orthotics to treat biomechanical imbalances, injuries, and illnesses of the feet. If you have bunions, arthritis, or other foot ailments that make it hard to find shoes that fit, your doctor can refer you to an orthotist or pedorthist.

COMMON FOOT PROBLEMS

Arthritis

Arthritis is a disease characterized by inflammation of the cartilage and lining of the joints. When arthritis occurs in your feet, the joints of your feet can become swollen, stiff, and painful.

If left untreated, arthritis can be very disabling, and in severe cases it can cause deformity in the feet. Some people suffer from recurring short episodes of arthritis; for others, arthritis is a chronic condition that requires constant treatment.

WHAT CAUSES ARTHRITIS?

Of the many different types of arthritis, osteoarthritis, rheumatoid arthritis, and gout are the most common.

• **Osteoarthritis** is a breakdown in joint cartilage caused by normal wear and tear or by a traumatic injury to the joint. Most common in women and men over the age of forty-five.

- **Rheumatoid arthritis** is a more serious form of the disease characterized by acute onset and alternating periods of symptoms and remissions, caused by inflammation of the tissue (called *synovium*) that lines the joint. Women are three to four times more likely than men to have rheumatoid arthritis; it often strikes between the ages of thirty and forty and can flare up again after age seventy.[3]

  Arthritis can also sometimes occur in young adults and children. Doctors think that rheumatoid arthritis might be caused by an immune system disorder. Foot deformities like hammertoes, claw toes, and bunions can be caused by arthritis, as can other common foot problems like neuromas, flat feet, calluses, and inflamed metatarsal joints. Likewise, hammertoes and bunions can result in arthritis. Other causes of arthritis include heredity, viral and bacterial infections, and drug reactions.

- **Gout** is caused by a buildup of uric acid crystals in the joint fluid. It is most common in men over the age of forty.

How do you know if you have arthritis?

Painful, stiff, red, and/or swollen joints can be a sign of arthritis. Sometimes people who have rheumatoid arthritis experience a hot sensation around the inflamed joint.

Why is arthritis so painful?

When a joint becomes damaged, fluid accumulates in the surrounding tissue, causing inflammation and pain. As with any foot injury, particularly one that impacts the biomechanics of the foot, weight bearing on a sore foot often increases the pain.

How do you prevent it?

It might not be possible to prevent arthritis, but you can take measures to keep your feet as healthy as possible:

- Exercise regularly.
- Wear comfortable shoes.

- Maintain a healthy weight.
- Eat a nutritious diet.
- Take vitamin and mineral supplements.
- Practice stretching and strengthening exercises to help you keep your feet in good shape.

How do you treat it?

Over-the-Counter Remedies

- Take aspirin or ibuprofen for inflammation and pain. Take with food to prevent upsetting the lining of your stomach. Follow the instructions on the bottle, and your doctor's instructions.

- If your foot is disfigured by arthritis, wearing more comfortable shoes can help relieve some of the pain. You may need the help of a podiatrist or pedorthist to find shoes and/or custom-made insoles that fit your feet.

Depending on the type and severity of your arthritis, your doctor might prescribe a variety of treatments, including physical therapy, anti-inflammatory medications, or orthotics or foot pads to be worn in your shoes. In some cases, if these treatments do not alleviate the problem, surgery might be necessary to repair the damaged joint.

Home Remedies

Foot soaks won't cure arthritis, but they can soothe aching feet. (See pages 24–25 for arthritis foot soaks.)

WHEN TO SEE A DOCTOR ABOUT ARTHRITIS

If you have sudden pain, notice swelling or redness around a joint, or if your foot has become too painful to walk on, see a doctor. Even if the pain isn't severe, you might want to see your doctor so that you get a correct diagnosis and learn what you can do to keep your joints healthy.

Athlete's Foot

A fungal skin infection that occurs between the toes, athlete's foot can spread to other parts of the foot. Skin problems are among the most common foot problems; more than 26 million Americans have athlete's foot, and almost half of them have had it for 10 years or longer.[4] Although 70 percent of adults experience athlete's foot at some time in their lives, it is most common in adults and teenagers, with men being four times more likely than women to contract the infection.[5]

WHAT CAUSES ATHLETE'S FOOT?

Warm, sweaty feet are prime targets for infections because fungus needs warm, moist conditions to grow. Many factors make people susceptible to athlete's foot:

- Wearing tight shoes and socks that prevent ventilation
- Walking barefoot in public locker rooms
- Fungal or bacterial infections

- Participating in sports and fitness activities that cause the feet to sweat
- Not drying feet and toes thoroughly after bathing
- Living in a hot climate

HOW DO YOU KNOW IF YOU HAVE ATHLETE'S FOOT?

The skin between and around the toes becomes itchy, scaly, and dry. In some cases, the skin develops painful cracks in between the toes. The skin can also become inflamed with small blisters. You may feel a burning sensation.

HOW DO YOU PREVENT IT?

There are many ways to reduce your chances of developing athlete's foot:

- Keep your feet dry. After bathing, make sure you dry your feet well. You may want to put some powder or cornstarch between your toes and in your shoes. There are many over-the-counter powders and sprays for feet and shoes that are designed to help combat moisture.

- Take off your shoes whenever possible to air out your feet and warm them in the sun.

- Change your socks often and wear white socks, which are cooler than dark socks. Although there are dyes in most socks, regardless of color, white socks have less dye and are therefore less irritating to the skin.

HOW DO YOU TREAT ATHLETE'S FOOT?

Your main goals in treating athlete's foot are to find relief from the itching, to heal the fungal infection, and to prevent bacteria from entering the body through the infected area. Replace your socks after a fungal infection to prevent reinfection, and if you wear your shoes without socks on, you might also want to replace your shoes.

Over-the-Counter Remedies

- Antifungal ointments, creams, sprays, and powder can help. Some of the widely available brands include: Lamisil AT, Dr. Scholl's, Mycelex, Tinactin, NP27, Lotramin AF, and Zeasorb. Follow the instructions on the package, and from your doctor.

- It's important to continue treating the infection until you're sure it's healed so that it doesn't come back again. Depending on the antifungal medicine you use, it may take one, two, or four weeks to get rid of the infection. The ointments will be more effective if you also continue to follow the preventive measures listed on pages 147–148.

Home Remedies

- Keep feet dry, and if you live in a warm climate, expose your feet to the sun at least once a day.

- Tea tree oil, having both antiseptic and antifungal properties, is an effective treatment for athlete's foot. Rub 1–2 drops into the affected area twice a day with a cotton ball or washcloth.[6]

- Soak: Add 2 tbsp of baking soda or epsom salt, 1–2 drops of lavender, and 2–4 drops of tea tree oil to a basin of warm water. Soak for 15–20 minutes. Dry feet thoroughly.

- Chamomile lotion, rubbed into the feet, helps soften dry, cracked skin. Add either fragrance-free lotion like Lubriderm or a carrier oil like sweet almond oil or jojoba oil to a 1-ounce bottle, leaving space at the top to add more later. Add 3 drops of chamomile oil and 2 drops of lavender oil (which also has antiseptic and antifungal properties). Fill the rest of the bottle with your lotion or oil, and shake to disperse oils. Rub into feet twice daily, after soaking your feet.

WHEN TO SEE A DOCTOR ABOUT ATHLETE'S FOOT

Use antifungal ointment for as long as directed on the package; athlete's foot can reoccur if you stop treatment too soon. If you don't see improvement after four weeks, or if the infection becomes red, itchy, or swollen, see your doctor. Sometimes a bacterial infection can be mistaken for a fungal infection, or bacterial and fungal infections exist at the same time. In either case, you might need to use a different type of medicine.

Blisters

Blisters are soft, fluid-filled sacs that form between the top layers of skin. The skin covering a blister is usually clear, and the surrounding skin is red. A severe blister, called a blood blister, occurs when a blister fills up with blood. Blisters can form anywhere on the feet, and are most common on the ball of the feet, toes, and back of the heel.

WHAT CAUSES BLISTERS?

Too much friction or pressure on the skin. The friction heats up the area and causes the outer layers of the skin to separate and fill with fluid.

HOW DO YOU PREVENT THEM?

You can prevent blisters by reducing the amount of friction on the feet:

- Wear shoes that fit well and socks that absorb or wick moisture away from the feet.

- Wearing thick socks, rubbing petroleum jelly on hot spots, and using foot powder can also help prevent blisters from forming.

- Wear shoes during recreational activities; going barefoot can cause blisters.

How do you treat them?

Over-the-Counter Remedies

Blisters are very common, and many products at your local drugstore or supermarket can help protect your feet. **Caution:** If you have diabetes or circulatory problems, do not self-treat blisters; see your doctor.

- Cover your blister with a bandage, moleskin, or blister pad to protect it and reduce friction. It should go away after a few days.

- Try switching to another pair of shoes (or sandals) or wearing neoprene insoles to cushion your feet.

- If your blister is too large or too painful to walk on, you can drain it. Sterilize a needle by holding it under a flame for a few seconds, then wipe it off with alcohol or peroxide. Puncture the top layer of skin in a few places, keeping the skin intact. (It's important to leave the covering intact to prevent infection. If the top layer of skin does come off, especially in the case of a blood blister, you should use a chemically moist dressing, like DuoDERM or Sorbsan pads, to protect the underlying skin.) Let the liquid seep out of the blister, then apply antibiotic ointment and cover with a bandage or gauze. You can drain blood blisters if they become too painful, but use caution. If bright red blood comes out of the blister, see a doctor immediately or go to the emergency room.

Home Remedies

- *Blister soak:* Add 5 drops of geranium oil and 2 trays of ice to a basin of cold water. Soak your feet for 20 minutes. You can also soak your feet in cold tea for 30 minutes (see page 30 for tea soak recipe), or in warm water and epsom salt. **Caution:** Foot soaks are not recommended for people with diabetes or circulatory problems.

- Apply 1 drop of lavender oil to the blister. Cover with a bandage. Do not use lavender oil on broken skin, or after draining blister.

WHEN TO SEE A DOCTOR ABOUT BLISTERS

If your blister becomes infected, prevents you from enjoying your normal activities, or if you have a chronic problem with painful blisters, see a doctor. Frequent blisters might be the result of a biomechanical problem. If this is the case, your doctor might prescribe orthotics to help stabilize the motion of your feet.

Bunions

One of the most common foot problems, bunions affect more than 11 million adults in the United States.[7]

WHAT IS A BUNION?

A bunion is a deformity of the big toe joint. Over time, a large, protruding bump (of tissue or bone) forms at the base of the joint, and often the big toe moves inward toward the other toes, causing a misalignment of the big toe joint and of the second toe. Bunions can became inflamed and very painful.

If not treated, bunions can deform the entire foot, and in severe cases make standing and walking impossible. Smaller bunions, called bunionettes, can form on the little toe.

WHAT CAUSES BUNIONS?

- Heredity
- Biomechanical deficiencies in the feet, including arthritis, flat feet, low or fallen arches, and pronation
- Years of wearing ill-fitting shoes

Women are fifteen times more likely than men to develop bunions because they wear narrow, high-heeled, pointed shoes that place stress on the feet by forcing them into unnatural shapes.[8]

How do you know if you have bunions?

There are many symptoms that might indicate that you have a bunion: a big toe that has moved closer to your other toes, joint pain and swelling, a protruding bump on your foot at the base of your big toe (your shoes may eventually stretch to accommodate the deformity), overlapping toes, calluses, ingrown toenails, and neuromas.

How do you prevent bunions?

You can prevent bunions by taking good care of your feet:

- Wear comfortable shoes with good arch supports.
- Practice foot-specific stretching and strengthening exercises (see pages 85–115).
- Pay attention to any symptoms you might have, and see a doctor before your foot problem gets too big. It's always easier and more effective to treat a foot problem when it starts, which also leaves you with more treatment options.

How do you treat them?

Over-the-Counter Remedies

- Cushion bunions with moleskin or foam doughnut pads.
- Wear sandals that don't put pressure on the inflamed joint, and buy wider shoes.
- Elevate your feet a few times a day for 20 minutes.
- If you have a pair of old shoes that you wear only around the house, you can cut out a hole where the joint rubs against the shoe to take the pressure off the joint. You can also try wearing foam toe spacers between your toes.

Home Remedies

Sometimes soaking your feet or giving yourself a foot massage can give you temporary relief from aching feet. (See bunion soak on page 25.) You can also apply a bag of ice to your bunion twice a day for 15–20 minutes. (Diabetics should not soak or use ice.)

- Get a full-body massage, with extra attention paid to your feet, or ask a friend or partner to massage your feet. You can also give yourself a foot massage. (See pages 54–59 for massage instructions and page 35 for massage oil recipes.)

WHEN TO SEE A DOCTOR ABOUT YOUR BUNIONS

If your foot hurts, if you notice swelling, or if you have any of the symptoms listed on page 157, see a doctor. Your doctor might prescribe orthotics, physical therapy, anti-inflammatory medication or injections, or in severe cases, surgery.

Corns and Calluses

Corns and calluses are small areas of thickened dead skin that form on the feet. Calluses occur on the ball of the foot and heel, and corns form on or in between the toes. Both usually form over a joint. Ten percent of adults in the United States have corns, and 19 percent have calluses.[9]

What causes corns and calluses?

When repeated pressure or friction on areas of the foot is more than the foot's natural padding can withstand, corns and calluses form to protect the underlying bones.

Some of the common causes:

- Wearing high-heeled shoes, or any shoes that are too small or that force the foot into an unhealthy position
- Going barefoot for long periods of time
- Standing on your feet all day
- Pronation or other biomechanical problems that interfere with how the body's weight is distributed over the feet
- In some cases, corns and calluses are hereditary

How do you know if you have a corn or a callus?

- Corns are hard bumps of dead skin that form on the surfaces of toes. When corns form in the space between your toes, they are usually soft. Sometimes corns have hard cores in their centers that burrow into the skin; they can become painful and inflamed if not treated.

- Calluses are also hard dry bumps of dead skin, but they are found on the bottoms of the feet. Calluses can also have cores. When calluses become painful, they create a burning or aching sensation.

- Both corns and calluses can become very painful when the underlying bone or joint becomes inflamed.

How do you prevent them?

- Wear comfortable shoes that fit properly.
- Wear cushioning pads or neoprene insoles in your shoes.
- Work with your doctor to address whatever biomechanical problems your feet might have.

HOW DO YOU TREAT THEM?

The best way to prevent or treat corns and calluses is to reduce or eliminate the pressure and friction that cause them to form. It could take a few weeks, or up to a few months, for a corn or callus to shrink.

- Wear shoes or sandals that don't rub against your corns or calluses. Shoes with a roomy toe box will give your feet and toes more room and help prevent friction.

- Pad the corn or callus with a foam doughnut pad to reduce pressure on the area. You can also use foam padding to cushion the ball of the foot or a metatarsal pad to alleviate pressure. (Ask your doctor or physical therapist how to place a metatarsal pad.)

- Sand down corns and calluses with a pumice stone or file.

- Soften your skin with foot soaks and lotions.

Over-the-Counter Remedies

There are a variety of over-the-counter corn and callus treatments, but not all of them are effective or good for you. Avoid medicated corn and callus pads because they contain salicylic acid and/or other chemicals that can irritate the skin, especially the soft, healthy skin surrounding the corn/callus.

Caution: If you have diabetes, or circulatory problems, do not trim your corns or calluses or use any products containing salicylic acid; see a doctor for corn and callus treatment.

Home Remedies

The following routine not only helps provide some relief from corns and calluses, it's a great way to pamper your feet.

Caution: If you have diabetes, or circulatory problems, you should not soak feet in warm water or use a pumice stone; see your doctor for treatment.

1. Softening Foot Soak

   Corn/callus softener: Add 2 tbsp baking soda, 2 tbsp of olive oil, and 5 drops of chamomile oil to a basin of warm water. Soak for 15–20 minutes.

   To reduce swelling: Add 2 tbsp epsom salt to a basin of warm water. Soak for 15–20 minutes. You can add 5 drops of eucalyptus oil, or five drops of lavender.

   Pat feet dry with a towel.

2. Exfoliation

   Using a pumice stone, gently sand corns and calluses using a back-and-forth motion. Rinse feet with water and pat them dry with a towel. (See pedicure section, page 47, for more information about exfoliation, and read the instructions that come with your pumice stone.) Do not try to get rid of corns and calluses in one treatment. They should be scrubbed down in small increments over a period of time to prevent burning the skin.

3. Apply moisturizing cream or lotion to feet. You can buy foot lotion at the store or make the following corn lotion: Pour some fragrance-free lotion like Lubriderm or Eucerin into a 1-ounce bottle, leaving some room at the top. Add 3 drops of chamomile oil and 2 drops of lemon oil. Fill the rest of the bottle with lotion. Shake well.

   If you're applying lotion just before bedtime, put on a pair of socks to hold in the moisture.

WHEN TO SEE A DOCTOR ABOUT CORNS OR CALLUSES

If your corns or calluses are painful when you walk, or if over-the-counter and home treatments haven't given you relief, see a doctor. Your doctor may file the corn or callus off, or prescribe orthotics to correct biomechanical problems in your feet.

Dry Skin

Most adults experience patches of dry skin on their feet, especially around the heels.

WHAT IS DRY SKIN?

Dry skin is simply skin that needs hydrating. The soles of the feet have the thickest layers of dead skin on the body, and trying to keep them moisturized can be difficult.

WHAT CAUSES DRY SKIN?

- Loss of moisture through perspiration
- Pressure on feet from supporting weight of body

There are also several skin disorders that cause dry feet, including athlete's foot (itchy, burning fungal infection of skin), dermatitis (itchy, scaly red patches of skin), eczema (inflammation of the skin), keratinization (body produces excess keratin, a protein that prevents the skin from absorbing moisture), psoriasis (bumpy rash and scaly skin), and xeroderma (mild drying of the skin).

HOW DO YOU PREVENT IT?

The best way to prevent dry skin is to keep it hydrated. Drink at least eight glasses of water throughout the day, and follow these guidelines:

- Wash feet daily, using very mild soap. Bathing too often, bathing in very hot water, and using harsh soaps contributes to dry skin. Gently exfoliate the skin with a bath brush or pumice stone.

- After bathing pat your feet dry with a towel. Rubbing your skin with a towel dries the skin too much. It's okay to leave a bit of moisture on your feet, but do dry thoroughly between your toes.

- Apply moisturizing cream or lotion to feet after bathing to hold in moisture. You don't have to buy special foot lotion; hand and body lotions work fine. As a general rule creams are better than lotions at sealing moisture into the skin. Use a cream that contains alpha-hydroxy acids, which exfoliate the top layers of dead skin and help compact the remaining surface layers to form a seal that keeps moisture in the skin. It's important to apply cream after bathing to seal in moisture; applying alpha-hydroxy cream on a dry skin will only seal in the dryness.

- A great time to moisturize feet is right before bed. Wash your feet or soak them, then apply cream or lotion, and wear socks to help keep in moisture. Make sure that when you put on your socks you don't rub off the lotion.

How do you treat it?

- Apply moisturizing lotion or cream two or three times a day after soaking or wetting the feet. (**Note:** lotions do not add moisture to your feet; they seal the skin so that moisture remains in the skin.) Look for the most natural products that are free of dyes, perfumes, and other harsh chemicals that could irritate the skin.

- Use a mild, fragrance-free soap.

- Take your shoes and socks off when you're at home and give your feet some air.

- Using a humidifier in your home, especially in the bedroom, may help in preventing dry skin.

Over-the-Counter Remedies

Shopping for creams and lotions can be confusing because of all the fancy terms companies use to label their products. Here are the definitions of a few of the most common terms: *humectants* are ingredients in a lotion that attract water and keep it sealed in the top layer of skin, *alpha-hydroxy acids* are natural fruit acids commonly added to creams and lotions to help shed dead skin cells and seal moisture into the skin, *lanolin* is a type of humectant.

When buying skin care products, look for simple, pure, and effective.

- Dr. Bronner's Liquid Soap (use diluted) is a mild, pure soap that's good for bath, shower, and foot soaks.

- Lubriderm, Eucerin, Keri, Cetaphil, and Amlactin are all good creams and lotions, and many of them come in fragrance-free versions. Vaseline is another good product for sealing in moisture, and you can also try foot lotions made by Aveda, Aubrey Organics, Vaseline, Neutrogena, and other companies.

Home Remedies

Chamomile oil is good for softening dry skin.

- *Dry skin soak:* Add 2 tbsp baking soda, 2 tbsp of olive oil, 2 drops of chamomile oil, 1 drop of lavender oil, and 2 drops of geranium oil to a basin of warm water. Soak for 15 minutes. Pat dry with a towel and massage feet with a rich moisturizing cream.

- *Dry skin lotion:* Place some fragrance-free lotion in a 1-ounce bottle, leaving room at the top to add more later. Add 3 drops of chamomile oil and 2 drops of lavender oil. Fill the rest of the bottle with the lotion. Shake to disperse oils.

WHEN TO SEE A DOCTOR ABOUT DRY SKIN

Redness, itching, and changes in the skin (flaking, rashes, bumps) could indicate an infection. If your symptoms last more than a few days, or if your skin is so dry that it's cracking and bleeding, see your doctor. Cracked skin can increase your risk of contracting a bacterial or fungal infection.

Ingrown Toenails

Ingrown toenails is one of the most common and painful foot problems. An ingrown toenail generally occurs in the big toe, when one or both sides of the toenail grows into the skin surrounding it, resulting in redness, inflammation, and pain.

WHAT CAUSES INGROWN TOENAILS?

- Cutting toenails too short or with curved edges
- Wearing shoes that are too small
- Fungal and bacterial infections
- Biomechanical foot problems

HOW DO YOU PREVENT THEM?

- Cutting your toenails straight across is the most important thing you can do to avoid ingrown toenails. It's easier to cut a nail straight across if you make several small clips as you work your way from one side of the nail to the other.

Use good toenail clippers, and don't cut your nails too short. For smooth edges you can gently file the edges of the toenails.

- Gently clean under your nails and along the nail grooves regularly. Metal implements should not be used to clean these areas; they are too sharp and could break the skin that seals the nail to the nail bed, increasing your chance of infection. Instead, use an orange stick (a small wooden stick with one slanted edge). Soak the stick in water first to soften it, or wrap the tip in a small piece of cotton from a cotton ball.

- Don't wear tight socks or nylons, which constrict the feet and toes. Wear comfortable shoes that support your feet. If you do wear nylons, pull out the material in the toe area after you put them on to give your toes more space.

HOW DO YOU TREAT THEM?

- Wear sandals to reduce the pressure on your toes.

- Apply antibiotic ointment to soothe the irritation and reduce inflammation.

- Watch for signs of infection: swelling, discoloration of skin or nail pus. If you think your toe is infected, see a doctor. An infected toe can lead to a serious health problem like gangrene, especially if you have diabetes or poor circulation.

- Toenail retraining. Every day place a small piece of cotton from a cotton ball into the space between your nail and skin (use a new piece of cotton every day), and eventually your toenail will grow around the cotton. Ask your doctor to instruction you in toenail retraining.

Over-the-Counter Remedies

Antibiotic ointments and sprays can be found in the foot care section of your local drugstore.

Home Remedies

Try a soothing foot soak to soften your feet and reduce inflammation: Add 2 tbsp baking soda or epsom salt to a basin of warm water. You can also add 3 drops of lavender oil and 2 drops of tea tree oil. Soak for 15–20 minutes.

WHEN TO SEE A DOCTOR ABOUT INGROWN TOENAILS

If the pain and inflammation don't decrease or go away within a few days, or if the toe looks infected, see a doctor.

Nail Fungus

Nail fungus is a fungal infection of the toenails. As common as athlete's foot, toenail fungus affects more than 5 percent of Americans (and 20–30 percent of older Americans).[10] Like athlete's foot, toenail fungus is more common in men than in women.[11]

WHAT CAUSES NAIL FUNGUS?

- Fungus under the toenails begins to eat away the nails

HOW DO YOU KNOW IF YOU HAVE IT?

A variety of symptoms may indicate a fungal toenail infection:

- Discolored toenail (nails might turn white, yellow, green, brown, or gray)
- Misshapen nail
- White spots on surface of nail and/or nail surface becomes rough, bumpy
- Nail becomes separated from nail bed
- Thickened nail

HOW DO YOU PREVENT IT?

- Wear shoes that fit well and that allow your feet to breathe.
- Wear thick white socks, and change them at least once a day.
- After bathing, completely dry feet and in between toes.

How do you treat it?

To determine whether your nail infection is fungal or bacterial, see your doctor to get an accurate diagnosis and treatment plan. Infections usually require prescription medication. A fungal nail infection can be very difficult to cure, and if not treated quickly, can spread to other nails.

Fungus can live in your shoes and socks, so once you've been treated for the infection, you will want to replace your shoes and socks to prevent reinfection.

Over-the-Counter Remedies

Your doctor might suggest the following as a first line of defense:

- Apply antifungal cream to infected area.
- Spray the insides of your shoes with antifungal spray.

Home Remedies

- Apply 1 drop of tea tree oil to infected area twice a day.
- Nail soak: Add 3 drops of tea tree oil and 2 drops of lavender oil to a basin of warm water. Soak for 15–20 minutes. Dry feet, and between toes, thoroughly.
- Do not wear nail polish if you have toenail fungus. The polish can seal in the fungus. Wait until your infection has healed completely before using polish again.

WHEN TO SEE A DOCTOR ABOUT NAIL FUNGUS

If your condition has not improved within a month, go back to your doctor. She/he might need to prescribe an oral antifungal medicine.

Smelly Feet

Also called bromhidrosis, smelly feet plague 38 million adults in America.[12] Each foot contains 250,000 sweat glands and produces up to a cup of sweat a day. For people who exercise and play sports regularly, the feet can produce even more sweat. Men suffer from smelly feet more often than women.

WHAT CAUSES SMELLY FEET?

Sweat is your body's natural way of controlling body temperature, but for some people, sweaty feet can turn into stinky feet. Smelly feet can be caused by a variety of factors, alone or in combination:

- Sweat from your feet combining with bacteria
- Wearing shoes with poor ventilation
- Excessive sweating caused by vigorous exercise or nervousness
- Abnormal or damaged nerves overstimulating the foot's sweat glands to produce excessive amounts of sweat

How do you prevent them?

- Change socks and shoes often.
- Alternate wearing a few different pairs of shoes during the week so that each day, at least one pair has 24 hours to air-dry.
- Wear white cotton or wool socks (white socks have less dye in them and are less irritating to the skin).
- Wear shoes made out of materials like leather or suede that allow your feet to breathe. Avoid rubber-soled shoes; only wear athletic shoes when exercising.
- Wash feet often, and dry them meticulously. You might want to try using antibacterial soap.

How do you treat them?

Treating smelly feet is important not only for your social life but to prevent other foot problems. Excessive moisture can increase your chances of getting blisters or athlete's foot. Your first step in treatment is to follow the prevention tips. You

might also find that some over-the-counter products help reduce or eliminate your odor problem.

Over-the-Counter Remedies

- Deodorant products formulated for feet can help reduce
  foot odor.
- Antiperspirant products formulated for feet can prevent
  feet from sweating.
- Foot powder can be used on feet and in shoes.

Home Remedies

See page 30 for smelly feet and sweaty feet soaks and sprays.

WHEN TO SEE A DOCTOR ABOUT SMELLY FEET

If nothing seems to reduce or eliminate your odor problem, or
if your sweating is so severe that your soggy socks are causing

blisters on your feet, see your doctor. In rare cases, she/he might prescribe a medication to block your nerves from stimulating the sweat glands in your feet. Surgery on those nerves is a last resort.

Swollen Feet

Swollen feet are a common occurrence after sitting or standing for long periods of time.

WHAT CAUSES SWOLLEN FEET?

- Injury or trauma to the foot
- Other foot problems like arthritis, bunions, and hammer-toes
- Sitting or standing for long periods of time
- Pregnancy

How do you prevent them?

- If you're at work, take a quick break every hour and walk around for a few minutes. You can also keep a wooden foot roller or other foot massage implements under your desk. Roll your feet across them a few times an hour.

- If you're on a long plane ride, drink a lot of water and walk around for a few minutes at least every hour. Wear boots or shoes that have a lot of room in them; if you take off your shoes during the flight, your feet will swell and your shoes will feel tight when you put them back on after several hours. Give yourself mini foot massages several times throughout the flight.

- If you're pregnant, your body's weight-bearing stance will change to accommodate the weight of the baby, so it's important to wear supportive shoes that have good shock absorption. It's common for women's feet to expand during pregnancy. You may find that during and after your pregnancy you need to go up one-half to one shoe size.

How do you treat them?

Over-the-Counter Remedies

Take aspirin or ibuprofen for inflammation and pain. Take with food to prevent upsetting the lining of your stomach. Follow the instructions on the bottle, and your doctor's instructions.

Health note: In some people, ibuprofen can cause swollen feet. Check with your doctor to find out which treatment is best for you. If you are pregnant, consult with your doctor before taking ibuprofen or aspirin or trying any of the home remedies.

Home Remedies

- At the end of the day, rest for 15–20 minutes with your feet up (lie down and place two pillows under your feet to raise them above the heart).

- Soak your feet in warm water and epsom salt, and add 3–5 drops of the following oils: lavender, eucalyptus, peppermint, or rosemary. (See page 7 for soak recipes.) If your feet are swollen from injury or an illness like arthritis or bunions, a cold foot soak might feel better.

Health note: If you have diabetes, do not soak or apply iceto your feet. If you are pregnant, consult your doctor before using essential oils.

- Massage your feet. Add one of the essential oils recommended for soaks to massage oil or to fragrance-free lotion. (See page 33 for lotion recipes.)

WHEN TO SEE A DOCTOR ABOUT SWOLLEN FEET

If your swelling occurs after an injury or trauma, doesn't respond to ice or ibuprofen, or if you have a chronic problem with swollen feet or have diabetes or a circulatory problem, see a doctor immediately.

Diabetes

Diabetic foot care might not be a concern for you, but it's worthwhile to understand a little bit about the special foot care needs of diabetics, since many of us have, or will have, older family members with diabetes. The preventive care information listed here, where applicable, can also be useful for older adults.

WHAT IS DIABETES?

Sixteen million people in the United States have diabetes, and almost 800,000 are diagnosed each year.[13] And one in five diabetics who check into a hospital do so for foot problems.[14]

People with diabetes, particularly older people, need to be aware that the complications of their disease can make ordinary foot problems dangerous.

WHAT CAUSES DIABETIC FOOT PROBLEMS?

The primary cause of most diabetic foot problems is neuropathy, a gradual loss of nerve function in the feet, and sometimes in the legs. Neuropathy may cause a variety of sensations in the feet—numbness, tingling, burning, shooting pain, and/or a pins-and-needles feeling. Neuropathy also causes a reduction or an absence of pain in the feet (also making it difficult for you to distinguish between hot and cold sensations), which means that simple foot problems like corns, blisters, or small cuts can go unnoticed until they become infected.

Because diabetes also impairs circulation to the feet, a minor infection can quickly become a major health complication because the feet don't receive the necessary blood supply to nourish tissues and heal wounds. In a diabetic, an open sore or ulcer can develop into a deep wound and even spread internally to underlying tissues and bones. In the worst cases, foot infections can become so severe that the infected limb must be amputated. According to the American Diabetic Association, there are 67,000 lower limb amputations in the United States a year that can be attributed to diabetic foot complications. Fifty to 70 percent of all foot amputations in the United States are in diabetic patients with insufficient blood flow or infection.[14] In most cases, though, good preventive care can keep your feet healthy.

One of the most serious foot problems of diabetics is a bone injury called "Charcot foot." In a Charcot foot, foot or ankle bones can become dislocated or fractured for no apparent reason, or as a result of a minor injury. This condition can cause the arch of the foot to collapse or other deformities.

HOW DO YOU KNOW IF YOU HAVE DIABETIC FOOT PROBLEMS?

Only a doctor can diagnose diabetes. If you are diabetic, you need to take good care of your feet. Watch for symptoms like swelling, redness, blisters, and ingrown toenails, and follow the prevention tips listed on the following pages. Have your doctor check your feet at least twice a year (more often if you are prone to foot problems).

The longer you have had diabetes, the more your chance of developing neuropathy increases. Because you may not notice the gradual loss of sensation in your foot, you and your doctor should pay close attention to any changes in your feet. Again, the key health risk diabetics face is developing ulcers or other vascular problems that could lead to foot amputation.

How do you prevent them?

You can't prevent neuropathy from occurring, but there are many things you can do every day to prevent foot problems.

Stay healthy:

- Follow your doctor's instructions about foot care, nutrition, and exercise.
- Pay attention to your blood glucose levels, blood pressure, weight, and cholesterol levels. Keeping diabetes under control will help your body fight infections.
- Don't smoke or drink caffeine (both restrict blood vessels).
- Inspect your feet twice a day (have a friend, family member, or caregiver inspect them if you can't): look for blisters, swelling, redness, dryness, cuts, ingrown toenails, bruises, or any changes in your foot's shape or appearance.
- If you do have a foot problem, even if you think it's minor, see your doctor.

Take care of your feet:

- Wash your feet daily in lukewarm water with mild soap. Test the water temperature with your fingers or elbow to make sure it's not hot, or have a caregiver test the water temperature. Make sure you dry feet thoroughly, especially between the toes. **Caution:** Do not do any of the foot soaks, or other remedies, in this book—soaking is not good for diabetic feet.
- You can apply moisturizing lotion to your feet, but don't put lotion between your toes. Excess moisture between the toes can lead to infection.
- Cut toenails straight across to prevent ingrown toenails. If you need help cutting your toenails, have them trimmed by your doctor.
- If you have corns or calluses, which are very common in diabetics, do not use medicated pads, or other medicine, to get rid of them; those substances can burn the skin. You can use a file or pumice stone (on dry feet) to file down small calluses, but if they are very thick, have your doctor do it. Never try to cut corns or calluses yourself.

- Never use electric blankets, hot water bottles, or other devices to warm the feet. If your feet are cold, wear socks.
- Don't walk around barefoot; you could cut or burn your feet.

Shoes and socks:

- Wear comfortable white cotton socks that absorb moisture and allow your feet to breathe. White socks contain less dye than colored socks and are less irritating to the skin; they also make it easier to spot cuts or other problems that might cause the feet to bleed. Cotton sports socks are ideal because they are thick and comfortable. You can also buy special seamless socks made for diabetics.

- Do not wear nylons, tight socks, garters, or any other type of stocking that constricts your feet and lower legs. Your socks should not have any seams that rub against your feet or toes. Do not wear socks that have been mended.

- Wear comfortable and supportive shoes. You want to have enough room in your shoes to prevent rubbing or friction that could cause foot problems. Buy well-cushioned shoes made of breathable material, like leather. (See page 116 for information on how to buy shoes.) Ask your doctor to recommend a pedorthist who is specially trained to fit and modify shoes for people with diabetes, bunions, and other foot problems.

- Inspect your shoes before you wear them. Look for any tacks or pebbles that might be lodged in the soles, and make sure there are no pebbles or other objects inside your shoes.

- Change shoes and socks once a day.

HOW DO YOU TREAT THEM?

Because diabetic foot conditions can develop quickly, you need to see your doctor as soon as you notice a problem.

Your doctor may prescribe many treatments and/or medications to keep your diabetes under control and to maintain your foot health. These could include:

- Medication, nutritional counseling, and exercise
- Instructions on how to fit and buy shoes
- Custom-made orthotics to support and cushion the foot
- Antibiotics for infections
- Casting for Charcot foot condition

WHEN TO SEE A DOCTOR ABOUT DIABETIC FOOT PROBLEMS

You should have a primary care doctor who monitors your diabetes on a regular basis. It might be necessary for you to see additional health care providers to address your foot and health conditions, including a nutritionist, a certified diabetes educator, an endocrinologist, a diabetic nurse specialist, an orthopedic surgeon, a podiatrist, a pedorthist, and a vascular surgeon.

TOP CAUSES OF FOOT PAIN

Sometimes your feet just hurt. Heel pain, in particular, is one of the most common foot ailments, and 70 percent of the 2 million reported annual cases of heel pain are women.[15]

The following chart describes some common sites and causes of foot pain, as well as some commonly recommended treatments that might bring relief. Pain is your body's way of telling you that something is wrong. If these simple treatments don't help you, if you have an acute injury, or if your pain lasts more than a few days or stops you from doing what you want to do, see your doctor.

Location	Causes	Treatments[16]
Heel	Plantar fasciitis (inflammation of the plantar fascia), heel spurs, overuse injuries, arthritis, Haglund's deformity (bony protrusion on back of heel), Achilles tendonitis (pain in back of heel).	Take aspirin or ibuprofen for inflammation and pain; soak painful area in icy water (or apply ice pack) 2–3 times a day for 15–20 minutes; wear comfortable and supportive shoes; stretch calf muscles and Achilles tendon daily; roll tennis ball under arch to massage foot; warm up adequately when playing sports or dancing and increase training gradually; add heel pads, cushioned insoles, or custom-made orthotics to shoes; limit weight-bearing activities that cause pain. Wearing Birkenstock sandals has been shown to reduce heel pain in some people.[17]

Location	Causes	Treatments[18]
Arch	Plantar fasciitis, cramps.	Same treatments as heel pain, plus: soak feet in warm water to relieve cramps; have someone massage your feet, especially the arches.
Forefoot	Inflammation or injury to metatarsal joints, sesamoid bones, bunions, stress fractures, overuse injuries (common in runners and dancers), neuroma (inflammation of or tumor on one of the nerves or of the tissue surrounding the nerve) between the toes.	Same treatments as heel pain, plus: add a metatarsal pad to orthotics to support your metatarsal arch and relieve pressure on the metatarsal area.

Location	Causes	Treatments[18]
Ankle	Overuse, sprain, or fracture.	For acute injuries and swelling, doctors and physical therapists recommend the RICE treatment: *Rest* the injured foot, and limit weight-bearing activities. *Ice* the injured area for 20 minutes, 3–4 times a day. *Compression.* Wrap the injured area in an Ace bandage or gel pack. (Remove or loosen the wrap if swelling makes it too tight.) *Elevation.* Rest with your feet up (place two pillows under your injured foot to raise it above the heart) 3–4 times a day for 20 minutes.

Products for Foot Pain

Before you spend hundreds of dollars on custom-made orthotics or physical therapy, ask your doctor if over-the-counter
products might be appropriate for your foot problem. A study
done by the AOFAS showed that in 95 percent of the patients
tested, heel pain was improved by a combination of using over-
the-counter heel cushions and practicing regular stretching exercises. (See more about stretching in Chapter 5.) Sometimes
minor adjustments can produce the results you need.

Here are some products that can be helpful in addressing
minor foot problems:

- Anti-inflammatory drugs like ibuprofen or aspirin.
- Foot soaks (see page 19).
- Insoles and cushioning pads.

Sometimes adding padding and/or insoles to your shoes can
reduce or eliminate foot pain. Dr. Scholl's makes a variety of
foam and gel cushioning pads and insoles, as well as products

for corns, calluses, blisters, and ingrown toenails. Spenco and Sorbothane both make a wide range of cushioning and shock absorbing insoles (made out of foam rubber, gel, neoprene, and other synthetic materials) for dress, casual, and athletic shoes.

Silipos insoles and heel cups are made out of silicone, a dense gel-like substance that provides cushioning and shock absorption. Viscolas also makes several different types of heel pads and heel cups.

Birkenstock and Finn Comfort both make shoes and sandals that have contoured cork footbeds that support the arches and absorb shock. The shoe insoles can be removed, modified, and worn in other shoes as orthotic devices. Birkenstock also has a line of insoles (for use in non-Birkenstock shoes) designed to support the longitudinal and the metatarsal arches of the foot. Made out of cork and other natural materials, Birkenstock insoles and Finn Comfort footbeds are an ideal option for people with chemical sensitivities or allergies to the plastic used in many custom-made orthotics. A 1979 study done by podiatrists at the California College of Podiatric Medicine found that wearing Birkenstock sandals helped relieve heel pain in some of their patients.

- Exercise and stretch feet. (See page 85 for foot and ankle exercises and stretches.)

Glossary

AOFAS   The American Orthopaedic Foot and Ankle Society is an international professional medical organization of orthopedic surgeons who specialize in treating foot and ankle diseases, injuries, and problems. The AOFAS sponsors and conducts research, provides continuing education classes to its members, and promotes foot health through educational outreach programs. The AOFAS website is www.aofas.org.

APMA   The American Podiatric Medical Association is a professional organization for doctors of podiatric medicine (podiatrists). The APMA accredits podiatric colleges and residency programs, provides continuing medical education credits to its members, and promotes foot health through educational outreach programs. The APMA website is www.apma.org.

Bio-mechanical problems

Biomechanical problems occur when the way the body moves, due to muscle imbalances, injury, or a person's natural gait, causes injury. For example, some people's feet roll inward when they walk (pronation) and others' roll outward (supination). Both are considered biomechanical problems because the feet are not in optimal alignment to support the body's weight, which usually results in stress, strain, and injury in the foot, and in other parts of the body.

Exfoliate

To remove the surface layer of dead skin with gentle abrasion.

Insoles   Insoles make up the inside layer of a shoe, upon which the foot rests. Many shoes today are made with removable insoles so that they can be replaced when they wear out or if a more cushioned or supportive insole is needed. Many health care companies make cushioned insoles for athletic shoes, work boots, and dress shoes.

Metatarsal pad   A metatarsal pad is a small pad, usually made out of foam or gel, that provides support and cushioning to the metatarsal arch. It is generally placed on an orthotic at the area just behind the second metatarsal joint to alleviate the pain of metatarsalgia (irritation or inflammation of a metatarsal joint), a neuroma, or other forefoot problem.

Orthotics   Orthotics are custom-made insole devices worn in shoes to support and cushion the feet, and to correct biomechanical problems. A good orthotic matches the shape of the foot and positions it so that joints, muscles, and bones work together for optimal functioning.

Pronation See Biomechanical problems.

Resources

Arthritis Foundation
Atlanta, GA
404-872-7100, 800-283-7800

National Institute of Arthritis
and Musculoskeletal and Skin
Disease Information
Center Clearinghouse
Bethesda, MD
301-495-4484
www.nih.gov/niams

American Orthopaedic Foot
and Ankle Society (AOFAS)
Seattle, WA
800-235-4855
www.aofas.org

American Podiatric Medical
Association (APMA)
Bethesda, MD
800-275-2762
www.apma.org

American Diabetes Association (ADA)
Alexandria, VA
703-549-1500, 800-232-3472

National Diabetes Information Clearinghouse
Bethesda, MD
301-654-3327

National Shoe Retailers Association (NSRA)
Columbia, MD
410-381-8282,
800-673-8446
www.nsra.org

Pedorthic Footwear Association
Columbia, MD
410-381-1167,
800-673-8447
www.pedorthics.org

Product Guide

During the many months of researching and writing this book, I became obsessed with my feet, testing all sorts of shoes and fun foot care products. These are some of the products that made my feet feel great:

POTIONS, LOTIONS, SOAKS, AND SCRUBS

Burt's Bees, Inc.
Farmer's Market Coconut Foot Creme
Raleigh, NC
800-849-7112
www.burtsbees.com

The Body Shop
Peppermint Foot Lotion, Refreshing Foot Spray, Pumice Foot
Scrub, Peppermint Foot Fizzy
Burlingame, CA
800-263-9746
www.the-body-shop.com

EO
My Dogs Are Barking Foot Care Kit
Corte Madera, CA
800-570-3775
www.eoproducts.com

Aubrey Organics
Feet Relief Massage Cream, Natural Sports Rub Massage
Lotion, Neat Feet Foot Scrub
Tampa, FL
800-282-7394

Diamancel Files and Foot Patrol Exfoliating Foot Creme
blissout catalog
Brooklyn, NY
888-243-8825
www.blissworld.com

Ivy's Herbal Delights, LLC.
Scentsation Body Lotion, Multidimensional Body Creme,
Soul-Body Ginger Soak
800-947-5016
www.ivyshd.com

Dr. Singha's Mustard Bath
London, England
Distributed by Dr. Singha's Natural Therapeutics
Austin, TX
512-444-2862
www.drsingha.com

Dr. Hauschka Skin Care, Inc.
Sage Foot Bath and Neem
Nail Oil
Hatfield, MA
800-247-9907

ESSENTIAL OILS, CARRIER OILS, SALTS, AND HERBS

Gritman Pure Essential Oils
Friendswood, TX
281-996-0103
www.gritman.com

Aura Cacia
Weaverville, CA
800-437-3301
www.auracacia.com

210

Samara Botane
Oils, dried herbs, containers, and pre-mixed potions
Seattle, WA
206-282-4532, 800-782-4532
www.wingedseed.com

Zenith Supplies, Inc.
Oils, containers, foot massage toys
Seattle, WA
800-735-7214, 206-525-7997
www.zenithsupplies.com

The Herbalist
Dried herbs, salts
Seattle, WA
800-694-3727, 206-523-2600
www.theherbalist.com

Milk and Honey Inc.
Flexology Massage Balls, Thumb-ease thumb massagers
Santa Fe, NM
505-474-7799

Dr. Scholl's
Memphis, TN
www.drscholls.com

SHOES AND SOCKS

Rockport
Marlboro, MA
800-762-5767
www.rockport.com

Birkenstock
Novato, CA
800-761-1404
www.birkenstock.com

New Balance Athletic Shoe, Inc.
Boston, MA
800-253-7463
www.newbalance.com

ASICS TIGER Corporation
Irvine, CA
800-678-9435
www.asicstiger.com

Naked Feet
A division of Utopia Marketing, Inc.
West Palm Beach, FL
561-835-9998

Mephisto
Franklin, TN
888-637-4478
www.mephisto.com

Paul Green
Carpenteria, CA
800-736-1974

Finn Comfort USA
Think! USA
Newbury Park, CA
800-361-3466

Taryn Rose
Beverly Hills, CA
800-440-7673
www.tarynrose.com

Theresia
Keene, NH
800-805-5443

Wigwam
Wigwam Mills, Inc.
Sheboygan, WI
800-558-7760
www.wigwam.com

Thorlos
Statesville, NC
888-846-7567
www.thorlo.com

Ecco
Londonderry, NH
800-359-4399
www.ecco.com

EXERCISE EQUIPMENT

The Hygenic Corporation
Thera-Band exercise bands
Akron, OH
800-321-2135
www.thera-band.com

Orthopedic Physical Therapy Products (OPTP)
The Rock Board, Slant Board
Minneapolis, MN
800-367-7393
www.optp.com

Road Runner Sports
Multi-Slant Board, Dr. L Toe Stretcher
San Diego, CA
www.roadrunnersports.com
800-600-9945

HEEL PADS AND HEEL CUPS

Silipos
Niagara Falls, NY
800-229-4404
www.silipos.com

Viscolas
Soddy Daisy, TN
800-548-2694
www.viscolas.com

Notes

Chapter 1. Feet Don't Fail Me Now

1. APMA, AOFAS
2. American College of Foot and Ankle Surgeons
3. APMA and *Harvard Health Newsletter*
4. APMA, AOFAS
5. Birkenstock *(Roger's Corporation Newsletter)*
6. Healthwise Handbook, Group Health, and American College of Foot and Ankle Surgeons
7. APMA and *Runner's World* magazine

Chapter 4. Rub Some Life into Your Feet

1. Nicola Hall, *Reflexology: A Step-by-Step Guide.*

Chapter 5. Foot Fitness

My sources were the AOFAS; Chris Dormaier, yoga teacher; Wolfgang Brolley, physical therapist; Susan Grote, physical therapist.

Chapter 6. If the Shoe Fits

1. AOFAS
2. Foot Health Foundation of America
3. AOFAS
4. Birkenstock
5. AOFAS
6. *Runner's World* magazine, February 1999

Chapter 7. When Feet Go Bad

1. Dr. Scholl's
2. APMA
3. Healthwise Handbook, Group Health
4. *Health Magazine*, 1992, November/December
5. *Seattle Times* article, August 22, 1999

Notes

6. Valeria Worwood, *The Complete Book of Essential Oils & Aromatherapy*, *Chicago Tribune*
7. Dr. Scholl's
8. *The Foot and Ankle Sourcebook*, M. David Tremaine, M.D., and Elias M. Awad, Ph.D.
9. Dr. Scholl's
10. APMA
11. *The Foot and Ankle Sourcebook*, M. David Tremaine, M.D., and Elias M. Awad, Ph.D.
12. *Backpacker*, September 1998
13. AOFAS, American Diabetes Association (ADA)
14. ADA
15. AOFAS
16. AOFAS
17. AOFAS
18. California College of Podiatric Medicine

Index

Index

prevention of foot problems, 189; pumice stone warning, 163; salicylic acid warning, 163, 190; shoes and, 133, 191–92; socks and, 191, 192; symptoms in feet, 2, 188; treatment of foot problems, 192–93; warnings, 8, 154, 158, 190; when to see a doctor, 185, 189, 192, 193

Diamancel diamond foot files, 46, 162

Dr. Bonner's Liquid soap, 170

Dr. Hauschka's Neem Oil for Nails, 46

Dr. Scholl's: corn, callus, blister, and ingrown toenail remedies, 199; cushioning pads and insoles, 198; pedicure line, 46; survey, 137

Dr. Singha's Mustard Bath, 46

Emery boards, 45

EO's peppermint and lavender foot salts, 46

Epilepsy cautions, 17, 37, 138

Epsom salt: in basic soak, 21; benefits of, 9; Bunion soak, 25; Fancy foot scrub, 32; Foot soak for cranks, 28; Runner's soak, 28; Sleepy soak, 26; softening soak, 175

Essentials oils, 10–19; amounts, 19; in basic soak, 22; benefits of, 9; carrier oils for, 16; cautions (health notes), 17; dilutions, 16–17; direct application of, 18; fragrance (aromatherapy), 9, 10–11; grade, therapeutic, 11, 19; potions and lotions, scrubs, and sprays, 32–42; safety, storage, and mixing tips, 18–19, 33; types, 9–10, 11; warm water soaks, 11. *See also specific oils*

Eucalyptus oil (*Euclyptus globulus*), 10; Bunion soak, 25; corn/callus swelling, 164; Fancy foot lotion, 34; Fancy foot scrub, 32–33; Headache soak, 31; Pick-me-up spray, 41; properties and uses, 12, 55; rejuvenating soaks, 23; Smelly foot spray, 39; Sore feet soak, 29; Sore joints soak, 24–25

Eucerin, 34, 165, 170

Everyday spray, 40–41

Exercise: ankle, 85–86, *86,* 100–102, *100, 102,* 105–9, *105, 106, 107, 108;* calf and ankle strengthening, 95–100, *96, 98;* calf stretch, 89–91, *90, 91;* foot strengthening, 82, 94–95, 114; foot stretches, 82, 85–88, *87, 88,* 91–92, *91;* general fitness and, 81; health notes, 84–85, 92, 104, 109; plantar flexion/dorsiflexion, 93–94, *94;* ratings, 84; tips before you begin, 83–84; tips on exercises, 99, 109; toe exercises, 82, 103–4, *103, 104,* 110–15; walk in the sand, 115

Exfoliation, 47; alpha-hydroxy acids for, 168; corns and calluses, 164–65; file for, 49, 162; instructions for, 47–48; pumice for, 47, 162, 164–65; salt scrub, 48; sand basin for, 21; Walk in the sand, 115. *See also* Scrubs

Fancy foot: lotion, 33–34; oil, 35; scrub, 32–33; sprays, 36–42

Fatigue: essential oils for, 14, 55; mental, essential oils for, 14; My feet are killing me soaks, 29; reflexology for, 73; rejuvenating soaks, 23–24

INDEX

Index

Index

INDEX